The Country Doctor's Kitchen

1,267 Pantry Prescriptions and Refrigerator Remedies for Almost Every Health and Household Problem

Publisher's Note

The editors of FC&A have taken careful measures to ensure the accuracy and usefulness of the information in this book. While every attempt was made to assure accuracy, some Web sites, addresses, telephone numbers, and other information may have changed since printing.

This book is intended for general information only. It does not constitute medical advice or practice. We cannot guarantee the safety or effectiveness of any treatment or advice mentioned. Readers are urged to consult with their health care professionals and get their approval before undertaking therapies suggested by information in this book, keeping in mind that errors in the text may occur as in all publications and that new findings may supersede older information.

"The Lord is pleased with those who worship him and trust his love."

Psalms 147:11

FC&A Medical Publishing®
103 Clover Green
Peachtree City, GA 30269

Produced by the staff of FC&A

ISBN 978-1-935574-25-5

TABLE OF CONTENTS

Everyday smart living

Top tips for tension prevention

Super strategies to live long and strong

Simple steps to better living

Connect with others to heal body and mind

Best ways to beat fatigue and boost energy

Natural, low-cost secrets to a healthy home

Anti-aging tricks to look great and feel even better

Can't-miss body-slimming solutions

Sure-fire ways to defeat disease

Arthritis: super joint soothers

Cancer: smart ways to keep it at bay

Diabetes: fast fixes for blood sugar problems

Digestive disorders: terrific tummy tamers

Heart disease: tactics to keep your ticker in top shape

Osteoporosis: bone-building breakthroughs

Eye problems: see your way to clearer vision

Index 363

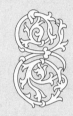

EVERYDAY
SMART
LIVING

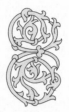

Top tips for tension prevention

6 serene secrets to soothing stress

You feel anxious or frustrated, you have trouble sleeping, and maybe you even get more colds or headaches than you once did. If this describes you, chronic stress may be affecting your health. Over time, this stress can raise your risk of heart attack, stroke, diabetes, depression, and even hair loss. Fortunately, relaxing and reducing stress doesn't have to be difficult. To start melting your stress away, try these refreshing tactics.

Start the day right. Getting ready in the morning can be miserable if you constantly struggle to keep things from tumbling off the counter. You may become even more frustrated if you frequently have to stop to hunt for items like your toothpaste or comb. These nagging hassles can jangle your nerves, make you run late, and leave you frazzled all day — all because you don't have enough space.

Fortunately, you can triple the storage space in your bathroom and de-stress your morning with this one simple solution. Pick up an inexpensive over-the-door shoe organizer with 24 clear plastic pockets. Hang it over the door, and fill it with your counter or sink clutter. If you still need more storage space, try one of these.

- Put wicker or plastic baskets in a bathroom cabinet to slide in and out, or try a lazy Susan. You can also hide stackable plastic baskets or bins behind a sink skirt.

- Tuck small items in a fishing tackle box, and decorate it to match your bathroom.

- Use muffin tins or plastic cutlery trays as homemade drawer organizers.

Change your mental radio station. If your brain were a radio, it would be tuned to Stress-FM, the "all stress, all the time" radio station. Obviously, you would enjoy listening to something else.

According to studies, people in hospital intensive care units and those preparing to have surgery or colonoscopies have successfully reduced their stress and anxiety by listening to music. Music also lowers your heart rate, blood pressure, and stress hormone levels. One study even found listening to music worked as well as the anxiety-relieving sedative midazolam.

To put this to work for you, choose comforting or soothing tunes you like. This can be classical music, instrumentals specifically labeled for relaxation, or old favorites from your high school years or other good times. You can even try country, pop, or jazz as long as it helps you relax and feel positive. Make time to listen to this kind of music every day, and let it take you away from your worries for a while.

Chew your stress out. Studies from Australia and Japan suggest chewing gum not only reduces stress and anxiety but your levels of stress hormones, too. Gum also may increase alertness while you chew it. Keep your favorite flavor of sugar-free gum on hand, and chew a piece when you feel your stress levels spiking upward. Aim to chew gum twice a day for five minutes or longer. In addition to reducing stress, this may also leave you with less mental fatigue and better spirits. Try to chew gum every day to keep the positive effects from wearing off.

Take a breather. A simple deep breathing technique can power up the relaxation centers in your brain. Instead of taking shallow breaths that make your chest rise and fall, take longer, deeper breaths that make your tummy rise and fall. This diaphragm breathing may help lower your heart rate and calm a region of the brain that controls anxiety. Practice doing this for several minutes every day — or any time you feel too tense.

Catch a whiff of relaxation. Everyone dreads getting shots, but a Korean study found that people who breathed in a lavender scent for five minutes were less stressed during their turn with the needle. They also experienced less pain. A scent that can do that probably will have no trouble over-powering your daily stress.

Many people enjoy using lavender-scented candles, soaps, lotions, or air fresheners to sweep away their anxiety, but research suggests these may produce unhealthy volatile oil compounds (VOCs). If you are concerned about VOCs, grow your own fresh lavender in a sun-drenched spot, or buy all-natural lavender tea bags.

Release tension in minutes. When you're under stress, your muscles tighten, and your body becomes as tense as a tightly coiled spring. Progressive muscle relaxation (PMR) is an easy way to relax your muscles and your mind in just a few minutes. It has even worked for people hospitalized with chronic obstructive pulmonary disease.

To do PMR, you start by relaxing the muscles in your toes and work your way up, gradually relaxing one group of muscles at a time, until you reach the top of your head. If you prefer, you can start with your head and work your way down. To watch a relaxing five-minute video that guides you through PMR, visit the Chronic Pain Association's website at *www.theacpa.org*, and click the link for Relaxation Guide.

Another relaxation exercise called focused attention may also help. In fact, it's so powerful it has even helped treat an anxiety disorder. To learn how to do this exercise, see "Surprising ways to manage chronic pain" in the chapter *Super strategies to live long and strong.*

Enjoy a double-duty defense against stress

Playing Wii Fit video games with your grandchildren — now that's a fun way to beat stress. And while you play, you're defending yourself against heart disease, colds, and other medical problems as well. Here's why.

Stress raises your body's level of cortisol — the fight or flight hormone — but that's not all bad because cortisol also regulates inflammation. Unfortunately, repeated floods of cortisol from stress may wear out your body's ability to respond to cortisol correctly, so your power to control inflammation wears away, too. As bouts of inflammation grow worse and last longer, they can trigger problems that cause heart attacks, diabetes, cold symptoms, or other health concerns.

To prevent this, you need a stress reliever that also fights inflammation. Exercise is the perfect remedy. Try activities like dancing, gardening, tai chi, yoga, exercise classes, or the fun-for-all-ages Wii Fit.

Make the most of your produce dollars

Some people avoid fresh produce because it goes bad before they finish eating what they bought. Others worry about news stories that have linked fresh fruits and vegetables to food poisoning and pesticide content. But study after study suggests eating that produce helps you live longer and prevent major health problems. So instead of eliminating produce from your grocery list, use these supermarket tips to keep it fresh and protect yourself from food poisoning and pesticides.

Enjoy the same nutrition for less

Don't be tempted by those out-of-season apples from New Zealand or cherries from Chile. The longer produce spends traveling, the more nutrients it loses. You may pay less for equally, or even more, nutritious foods if you try produce from one of these sources.

- Canned or frozen foods aisle. These foods are packed when ripe but are less expensive than imported produce. One study funded by the Canned Food Alliance suggests canned foods may offer equal nutrition at a better price than fresh produce.

- In-season produce. When produce is in season, determine whether you can stretch the season by buying it in bulk. Soup vegetables can be dried for off-season use. Apples can be dehydrated, too. And foods like carrots and cabbage may keep for two months if stored properly in the refrigerator.

Keep salad from going bad. Try these clever tricks to avoid waste, make your salads last up to several days longer, and save lots of money on produce.

- For a homemade salad, choose sog-resistant lettuce like romaine or red leaf.

- Tear lettuce into pieces and wash. Dry with either a salad spinner or a combination of colander and paper towels.

Store the lettuce in a bowl with a paper towel to absorb moisture, and cover with plastic wrap. Change the paper towel daily to keep the lettuce from becoming soggy and inedible.

- Moisture from certain salad ingredients is another source of sogginess and wilting, so don't store lettuce in the same container as "wet" ingredients like cut tomatoes, cucumbers, artichoke hearts, dressing, croutons or proteins like egg, chicken, and cheese. Some people say they have successfully stored lettuce with dry ingredients such as whole grape tomatoes, carrots, broccoli, onion, or radishes, but this may not work in all situations.

- Wash and prepare other salad ingredients the same day you prepare the lettuce. Use a salad spinner or paper towels to dry wet vegetables. Some also recommend leaving boiled eggs and wet fruits like tomatoes and oranges whole until you use them. Consider substituting grape tomatoes or dried fruit for wet fruits when appropriate.

- For best results, store each ingredient separately, and assemble the salad shortly before eating or packing it for lunch. This should only take a minute or two for each serving. Never add dressing until time to eat.

Make celery and carrots last longer. The trouble with celery is you always have to buy more than you need. Try this trick to keep celery fresh for weeks. Trim the ends of the celery, and wash and dry each stalk. Wrap the celery in dry paper towels, tuck in a plastic bag, and place in the refrigerator crisper drawer. Tipbusters.com put this to the test, and their celery was still crisp and free of browning after nearly four weeks.

To help carrots last longer, trim off their tops, and slip them in an open or perforated plastic bag.

Shop smart and stop food poisoning. Between 1990 and 2006, more than 25,000 cases of food poisoning were caused by five foods — potatoes, tomatoes, sprouts, berries, and leafy greens like spinach. Remember these foods so you'll take extra care when you choose and prepare them. But use the following guidelines for all the produce you buy.

- Only pick fruits and vegetables that are not bruised or damaged.

- Bag produce separately from meat, seafood, or poultry products. If you carry your groceries home in reusable grocery tote bags, always wash them between uses.

- Only buy bagged greens or pre-cut produce that is refrigerated or tucked into a bed of ice.

- Wash all fruits and vegetables under cold running water just before using them, even organic produce and items you plan to peel. Dry with a clean paper towel.

- Scrub melons, cucumbers, and other firm produce with a clean produce brush.

Enjoy fresh and clean fruits and veggies. The last thing you want on your farm-fresh produce is a farm-fresh coating of pesticides or chemicals. So buy locally grown produce when it is in season because it may have fewer pesticides. Check out farmers markets in your area if you can't find locally grown produce at your supermarket.

Also consider buying organic versions of those fruits and vegetables that have the highest levels of pesticides. This "worst offenders" list includes apples, bell peppers, celery, cherries, nectarines, peaches, pears, potatoes, raspberries, spinach, and strawberries as well as grapes grown outside the United States.

How you wash your produce can make a difference as well. Wash all produce under cold, running water. If you're concerned you may not remove enough pesticide, don't fret. Just mix three parts water with one part vinegar, and pour into a spray bottle. This all-natural recipe can help wash away the harmful toxic chemicals and pesticides hidden on grocery produce that plain water just can't. For even more protection, throw out the outer leaves of lettuce and cabbage heads before you wash or rinse them. Scrubbing firmer fruits and veggies like apples or potatoes while you rinse them can also help.

Pick like a pro. Think you don't know how to pick the best fruit? You will when you use these tips.

Fruit	Best season to buy	Secrets to perfect picking
apples	autumn	Pick firm, smooth-skinned apples with no bruises or soft spots. Rubbing your thumb across the skin should not cause wrinkling.
berries	summer	Choose firm berries without blemishes. Tilt the container to check berries in the bottom. Ripe blueberries have a "bloom" that resembles a dusting of white on the berries.
cantaloupe	summer	Check for a hint of yellow throughout the rind and a sweet cantaloupe smell.
oranges	winter	Look for full coloring with no green areas, firmness, and a fruit that is heavy for its size.
peaches and nectarines	summer	Avoid very hard or soft fruits and those with bruises. Check for a sweet, peachy aroma.
tomatoes	summer	Choose shiny, brightly colored tomatoes with a sweet, earthy scent and no cuts or bruises.
watermelons	summer	Look for a watermelon with a creamy or yellow underside and no stem attached. Heft two equal-sized melons from the bin and choose the heavier one.

5 ways to ease stress at the supermarket

Budget-busting prices, misleading labels, and battered produce are just a few of the things that make grocery shopping stressful. But that doesn't mean you are stuck with them. Use these tips to help ease supermarket stress, save money, and protect your health.

Get rid of your pile of coupons. You can spend less on groceries without ever fumbling with a pile of paper coupons again. Use electronic coupons instead. Just store them on your grocer's loyalty card or on your smartphone. Here's how.

- Visit your grocer's website to download coupons to your loyalty card. You may also find coupons for your favorite grocery store on one of these sites — *zavers.com, cellfire.com,* and *shortcuts.com*. Downloaded coupons are automatically deducted from your bill when you swipe your loyalty card at the checkout.

- Download coupons to your smartphone from the website or smartphone app of your grocer or favorite product manufacturers. While shopping, watch for smartphone codes on displays or packages of products you buy. Scan them with your smartphone to pick up discounts when you check out.

Make friends with the staff. You use coupons and check the store's weekly flyer, but you still may miss some bargains and opportunities. Fortunately, the supermarket staff has the inside scoop on these. Get to know them, and ask questions. For example, produce clerks can tell you when the next shipment of your favorite apples will arrive, so you can buy them fresh before they're damaged by frequent handling. The store manager or the customer service desk staff can answer questions about coupon policies, upcoming promotions, unadvertised discounts, new ways to save money, and more.

Understand unit pricing. In some stores, the shelf price tags not only display the price of the product but its per unit price, too. Comparing unit prices is the best way to tell which products give you the best deal. For example, if an 8-ounce can of tomato sauce has a unit price of $0.08 and the 16-ounce can is $0.06, you know the larger can will give you more for your money. Of course, that's only true if you can use it all before it goes bad.

Unfortunately, in many states these labels are voluntary and don't follow any common standard. One product may be unit priced by the ounce, while its competitor is priced by the pound. And, in at least one case, investigators discovered the unit prices of some stores were not accurate.

If you suspect the unit prices might be wrong, you can easily check them with your calculator. For a 32-ounce bottle of juice costing $4.50, divide the cost by 32 to get the price per ounce, in this case $0.14. If the products you're comparing don't have equal measures — say, ounces vs. pounds — you'll have to do a little more math to level them out.

Know what ingredients to look out for. Reading labels and ingredient lists is a good way to eat healthy. One benefit of eating healthy foods is it may help keep your cholesterol levels down so you can avoid taking prescription drugs.

But do you know the one word on food labels you should avoid like the plague? Surprisingly, it's not fat. The word is "hydrogenated," and you should always check the ingredient list to see if it's there. Why? The term "partially hydrogenated" means the product contains trans fats. These trans fats raise your "bad" LDL cholesterol and lower your "good" HDL cholesterol — exactly what you don't want.

Another term you may see is "fully hydrogenated." These oils basically turn into saturated fats and contain no trans fats so many companies are using them to replace partially hydrogenated fats. But they may not be much better because some are combined with vegetable oils, resulting in "interesterified" fats, which may have their own health consequences. One small study has suggested that inter-esterified fats may lower HDL cholesterol, although more research is needed.

Meanwhile, play it safe. Product labels and ingredient lists may not tell you when fully hydrogenated fats are part of interesterified fats, so avoid any product with "hydrogenated" in its ingredient list.

Avoid "health foods" that can kill you. That "healthy and natural" box of crackers may not be good for you, even if it promises "trans fat free" or "no cholesterol" on the package. Here's what product manufacturer's don't want you to know about dangerously misleading labels.

Trans fat free does not guarantee the product has no trans fats. FDA guidelines allow this claim for products with up to one-half gram of trans fat per serving. But if a serving is five crackers and you eat 20, you have eaten 2 grams of trans fats. The Institute of Medicine says even the smallest amounts of trans fats are not safe, and studies suggest these fats may raise your risk of heart disease, diabetes, and some cancers.

The "no cholesterol" label has similar problems. FDA guide-lines allow this claim for products with up to 2 milligrams of cholesterol and 2 grams of saturated fat per serving as well as unlimited amounts of trans fats.

Don't let these faulty claims guide your buying decisions. Instead, be your own food inspector. Examine the Nutrition Facts label to make sure the product has no saturated fats or trans fats. Then scour the ingredient list to be sure the word hydrogenated is not lurking there, and check the serving size to see how closely it matches the amount you will eat. This helps limit trans fats and saturated fats so you can stay healthy for a long time to come.

Save yourself from germ-infested carts

Would you put food on a toilet seat? When you place it in a grocery cart, you might as well be. A University of Arizona study found that nearly three out of four grocery carts may carry germs you normally find in a toilet. What's more, half the carts examined in the study carried the food poisoning bug *E. coli.*

Fortunately, many supermarkets now offer disinfectant wipes near the carts. Use one to wipe the cart handle before you shop. And don't place any food in the fold-out basket near the cart handle unless that food will be cooked.

If you must put food in the basket, bag it first — just in case leaky meat packages or leaky diapers were in the basket before you came along. Discard the bag as soon as you get home, and wash your hands thoroughly.

Amazing health-boosting kitchen tricks

You want to eat right so you can live long and keep your good health, but the nutrition guidelines seem harder to understand than your taxes. Just remember, you don't have to master them all at once. In fact, you can even make your efforts in the kitchen fun and delicious. Start with these clever ideas.

Use a greener fat cleaner. You used a cheaper cut of beef in your soup to save money, and now extra fat is pooling on the soup's surface. That extra fat is bad for both your health and your trim figure. Fortunately, you already have a free fat remover in your refrigerator — a lettuce leaf. Drop this grease magnet into your soup or chili during cooking. Simply remove the leaf before serving, and you have removed unwanted fat.

Savor a super soup. Use summer's bounty of fresh tomatoes to whip up a tangy soup bursting with flavor and health benefits. This soup may help lower "bad" cholesterol, boost a disease-fighting compound in your body, and keep you cool when it's 90 degrees in the shade.

What is this incredible soup? It's gazpacho, that mouth-watering combination of tomatoes and savory ingredients like garlic, onions, vinegar, olive oil, cucumbers, and bell peppers. The tomatoes not only taste good, they also serve up a powerful disease-fighter called lycopene. Research shows 25 milligrams of lycopene may be enough to lower LDL cholesterol by 10 percent.

Of course, one serving of gazpacho won't give you that much lycopene, but you have plenty of other high-lycopene foods to choose from. These include salsa, tomato juice, pasta sauce, tomato-based soups, plain or vegetarian baked beans, barbecue sauce, and foods made with tomato paste, tomato puree, or even ketchup. In the fight against heart disease, stroke, and high blood pressure, eating this food in any form is a great thing to do. After all, research suggests lycopene's powers include these special abilities:

- thins your blood and prevents clots so you're less likely to have a heart attack or stroke. In fact, one study found that men with the lowest blood levels of lycopene have a higher risk of a heart attack or stroke.

- lowers blood pressure. Researchers discovered that 7 ounces of raw tomato a day lowered blood pressure in people with diabetes in just eight weeks.

- helps fight inflammation.

Studies also suggest that eating tomatoes can lower your danger of osteoporosis, some cancers, and skin damage from the sun. Just remember to eat a little fat with your lycopene-rich foods. Fats like the olive oil in a gazpacho or pasta dish help you absorb more health-defending lycopene.

Enjoy a richer mayo. Use the paddle attachment on your mixer to make avocado puree, and mix in a splash of lemon juice for each avocado. Use this puree to replace mayonnaise in sandwiches and tuna salad. Even if you use low-calorie mayonnaise, switching to an equal amount of avocado puree cuts calories, sodium, and fat. You are also rewarded with more protein, fiber, and nutrients, plus a creamy twist of flavor.

Switch from tasteless to tantalizing. Try this if beans have become boring. Add some chopped garlic to the soaking water for dried beans. The garlic flavor will sneak into the beans, which not only tastes fabulous but also gives your beans a one-two punch against cancer. The fiber in beans helps prevent colon cancer, but eating cooked and raw garlic regularly may help slash your risk even more.

Yet that's not all garlic can do for you. Garlic supplements have been used to treat blood pressure, cholesterol, diabetes, and even the common cold. But check with your doctor before you try supplements or before eating more than six cloves of garlic a week. Garlic may not be safe for everyone. For example, garlic may be more risky for people who expect to have surgery or dental work soon and for those who take blood-thinning drugs like warfarin.

On the other hand, if your doctor approves, consider adding more raw garlic to your diet. Some people say they have fought off colds and other winter illnesses by regularly eating raw garlic rather than garlic supplements.

Just be sure you never eat raw garlic on an empty stomach or by itself. Instead, mince fresh, raw garlic and add it to your salad dressing, guacamole, or freshly made hummus. You can even add it to sandwiches for extra flavor. But start small, and add more garlic gradually to help avoid side effects like indigestion, gas, and diarrhea.

Sneaky way to enjoy more veggies

People will eat up to two more servings of vegetables a day if the vegetables are pureed and added to another dish, recent studies suggest. In many cases, the study participants could not taste the difference between a regular dish and one with extra vegetables.

To try this yourself, add pureed carrots to pasta sauce, slip pureed cauliflower into macaroni and cheese, or mix pureed lentils into meatloaf or hamburger patties. Pureed, shredded, or finely diced vegetables can also be added to stews, soups, casseroles, lasagna, mashed potatoes, gravies, or sauces.

Puree vegetables ahead of time, freeze them, and experiment with different amounts and different vegetables in your favorite dishes. Good veggies to try include carrots, sweet potatoes, zucchini, spinach, peas, broccoli, or black beans. Just make sure you don't add a vegetable that turns your recipe an unappetizing color.

Cut baking fat with sweet substitutes. The next time you make a coffee cake, substitute half a mashed banana for each cup of oil. This subtracts fat and calories while adding fiber, potassium, and a yummy taste. For other baked goods, try fat-cutting substitutions like these.

- Replace half the fat with an equal amount of pumpkin puree to add extra flavor and color.

- Substitute an equal amount of unsweetened applesauce for the fat, and reduce the liquid ingredients a little to make up for the added moisture. Or try replacing just half the fats called for with an equal amount of applesauce.

- For extra fiber, replace the fat in chocolate baked goods with pureed prunes. If the fat you replace is an oil or other liquid, add a little extra milk or water.

Remember, using fruit substitutes will change the texture and taste of your baked goods, so you may have to experiment to find the proportions you like.

Turn cheap meats into deal-icious delights

Makeovers are popular for everything from people to homes. You can even give your cheap cuts of meat a makeover. Here's how to make them just as tempting as more expensive cuts and help take a bite out of your beef budget.

Try a not-so-ancient Chinese secret. Chinese restaurants use baking soda to make cheaper meats "fork-tender," but you can do this at home, too. Just follow these easy steps.

- Cut the meat into strips or cubes. Tenderizer only works where it makes contact with the meat, so it helps to have smaller pieces. Cut across the grain or meat fiber markings to make the beef even more tender.

- For meat that is still damp from recent thawing, sprinkle baking soda over it, and rub in thoroughly. If the meat is dry, make a paste of baking soda and water and rub that into the meat.

- Let the beef rest in a covered container in the refrigerator for a few hours.

- Rinse the baking soda off the meat.

- Pat dry with paper towels, and continue preparing the meat for your soup, stir fry, fajitas, stew, casserole, or other recipe.

Turn tough meat into velvet-soft morsels. Chinese cooking also uses a technique called velveting to tenderize meat. As with the baking soda method, you must cut meat into cubes or strips before you begin.

For 1 pound of meat, mix one egg white and one tablespoon of cornstarch in a bowl, and coat the beef with this mixture. Marinate the beef in a lidded container in the refrigerator for 20 to 30 minutes.

In either a wok or a 12- or 14-inch skillet, heat two cups of oil between 260 and 280 degrees. Check with a thermometer. Add the beef, and let cook for about 30 seconds. Remove the meat quickly and drain it. This tenderizes the meat but may not completely cook it. Finish cooking the beef with your other recipe ingredients.

Discover the downside of baking soda

At first, this sounds like a great tip from the Web — add baking soda to the pot to keep cauliflower white and crisp when you cook it. But experts say this does not work. In fact, baking soda is a little like Dr. Jekyll and Mr. Hyde. It can tenderize meat quite nicely, but it can also devastate your vegetable dishes in several ways.

Baking soda not only destroys health-building vitamins like vitamin C, it also makes your vegetables mushy, and turns cauliflower and other white vegetables a sickly yellow. If you have already experienced problems like these, stop using baking soda when you cook cauliflower. You may be amazed at how much better it turns out.

Tenderize meat in a hurry. When tenderizing meat at home will take more time than you can afford, consider this. If you are on good terms with the staff at your supermarket meat counter, pick a tough cut of meat, and ask the clerk to run it through the tenderizer for you.

Prevent bone-dry roasts. You can make a juicy roast every time by avoiding this common mistake. It's easy to let your pot roast dry out in the oven if you don't check to make sure the lid fits correctly. Moisture may escape if your pot lid does not seal perfectly, so cover the pot with aluminum foil, or crimp a ring of foil around the lid to perfect the seal. If that's not enough to make your roast tender, check the roast regularly and add more liquid, if needed.

Make beef healthier and tastier. Season beef with garlic, and you may be more likely to avoid hospital stays, prescription drugs, and early death. In fact, this single herb could help prevent the top three killers in America. Here's how.

- Fights heart disease. Crushing garlic forms a powerful health-promoting compound called allicin. Studies show allicin can help lower "bad" LDL cholesterol, total cholesterol, and triglycerides, three known contributors to heart disease. Garlic also helps lower high blood pressure, another risk factor for heart disease. In fact, even if you have already begun developing heart disease, garlic may help slow its progress.

- Prevents cancer. Years of studies suggest garlic lowers your risk of colon cancer. Eating moderate amounts ranging from several cloves a week to two cloves a day may help protect you from both colon and kidney cancers. Just be sure to talk to your doctor before eating more than one clove of garlic a day. It may not be safe if you take certain medications or expect to have surgery soon.

- Slashes stroke risk. Garlic has blood-thinning powers that help prevent blood clots. Not only does this lower your risk of heart problems but also your risk of stroke.

To enjoy these garlic benefits, you must crush the garlic and let it rest for 15 minutes before using it in cooking. What's more, always add garlic during the last few minutes of cooking. Add it any earlier, and garlic's valuable compounds and health benefits will be reduced or destroyed.

Rescue your recipe with clever substitutes

Run out of milk? Used the last onion? No sign of the baking powder? Discover these no-fail substitutes you should always keep in your pantry.

Ingredient	Amount	Substitute
baking powder, double acting	1 tsp	1/4 tsp baking soda, 1/2 tsp cream of tartar, 1/4 tsp cornstarch
brown sugar	1 cup	1 cup granulated sugar
butter	1 cup	7/8 cup oil with 1/2 tsp salt
buttermilk	1 cup	Take out 1 Tbsp milk and add 1 Tbsp of vinegar or lemon juice. Let stand 5 minutes. Or substitute powdered buttermilk. See package instructions for the right amount.
chocolate, unsweetened	1 ounce	3 Tbsp cocoa with 1 Tbsp butter or vegetable oil
cornstarch	1 Tbsp	2 Tbsp all-purpose flour
egg	1 large	1/2 tsp baking powder, 1 Tbsp vinegar and 1 Tbsp liquid (in baking)
garlic	1 small clove	1/8 tsp garlic powder or instant minced garlic
lemon zest (fresh grated lemon peel)	1 tsp	1/2 teaspoon lemon extract
milk, skim	1 cup	1/3 cup instant nonfat dry milk plus 7/8 cup water
milk, whole	1 cup	1/2 cup evaporated milk plus 1/2 cup water. Can substitute 1 cup fruit juice in baking.
onion	1 small	1 to 2 Tbsp instant minced onion or 1 tsp onion powder
white flour, all-purpose, self-rising	1 cup	1 cup all-purpose flour plus 1 1/4 tsp baking powder and 1/4 tsp salt
wine, red	any	equal amount of grape juice or cranberry juice
wine, white	any	equal amount of apple juice or white grape juice

10 sneaky ways to cut your utility bill

Live without electricity like the Amish, and you may save plenty of money on utility bills. But you also may be so miserable that you give it up before long. Instead, why not try "sneaky," nearly painless changes you may barely even notice. You could save yourself a bundle just by using these tips.

Dry your clothes faster. It's easy. Just add a clean, dry towel to the dryer. Some people say this trick reduced their drying time by 50 percent or more. Switch to line drying only, and you could save up to $45 a year. Try an outdoor clothesline, indoor bars, or indoor folding racks.

Water prized plants for free. Gallons of free water and significant water bill savings may be waiting for you if you have central heating and air conditioning or a window air conditioning unit. Both types of air conditioning use a drain line to remove water that condenses on the air conditioner coils.

If your drain line does not connect to the sewer, you can collect this water to irrigate plants in your home or yard. Amounts collected range anywhere from one quart to 50 gallons a day, depending on how much your air conditioner runs. Window air conditioners supply far less water than central air units, but you may still collect up to two gallons a day, enough to water houseplants or other container plants.

A five-gallon bucket may be big enough to collect the water from some air conditioners, but others may require a large, clean garbage can or rain barrel. Before you set this up, find out if local and state regulations allow you to use this water, and whether large collection hook-ups require an inspection.

Remember to use collected water within three days, or cover the inlet with mosquito screening to prevent mosquitoes from breeding in your water. Do not drink any water collected from your air conditioner. It's safe for plants, but not people.

Switch to cold rinse for cold cash. Set your washer to rinse with cold water. You could save up to $25 every year. You'll save even more if you do most of your washing in cold water as well.

Escape this money trap. The dryer lint trap is also a money trap. The more clogged it gets, the harder your dryer has to work to circulate air and dry clothes, and the more your power bill goes up. Clean the lint trap before every load to save that money.

Tame the kitchen energy hog. Your refrigerator can account for up to 10 percent of your electric bill. If the door seal or gasket is damaged or worn, warm, moist air seeps into the refrigerator. This forces your refrigerator to use more electricity to maintain the same temperature, so you pay a bigger electric bill because the refrigerator no longer works efficiently. That's reason enough to check the door seal regularly.

A newspaper or dollar bill can tell you whether your refrigerator is working efficiently. Open the refrigerator door, hold a dollar bill or single sheet of newspaper against the seal, and close the door on it. Gently try to pull the paper or bill out of the door without opening it. If the paper or bill comes away easily, you need to change your refrigerator gasket.

Slash heating dangers and costs. Problems with your heating system don't just cause higher electric bills. They can make you sick and even threaten your life. For example, furnace leaks or cracked heat exchangers can cause carbon monoxide poisoning, while mold and mildew growing in ducts or on air filters can lead to hay fever symptoms and bronchitis.

Fortunately, you only need to do two things to lower your heating costs, avoid high-priced furnace repairs, extend the life of your heating system, and reduce the amount of dangerous toxins in your home. Simply have your furnace or heating system serviced regularly, and change its air filters as often as the manufacturer's instructions recommend. This keeps you cozy, safe, and free from worries about big heating repair bills.

Scrap your screensaver. You may have heard that the screensaver on your desktop computer saves energy, but that's a myth. Turn off your screensaver, and adjust your power management settings so the monitor and computer power down when they're not in use. That change could save up to $75 a year.

Save at the sink. Everyone does it. You turn on the faucet and let it run until the water gets cold enough for what you need. But you don't have to keep adding to your water bill. Just keep a jug of cold water in the refrigerator, and use that whenever you need cold or chilled water.

To save even more money, remember this. The moment you turn the kitchen faucet lever to the hot position, your water heater starts heating even if you turn off the tap before the hot water reaches the faucet. Those pennies add up, so avoid pushing the lever to the hot position when you don't need hot water. Make sure you collect any cool water that runs while you wait for the hot water, and add it to your cold water jug in the refrigerator.

Plug your electricity leaks. Up to 10 percent of your household's electricity may be going to devices that are turned off. These include your television, microwave, cell phone charger, VCR, and even night lights. Each one draws a tiny amount of electricity 24 hours a day all year long, even when you are not using them. The cost of these tiny currents adds up quickly because the average household has 40 energy-leaking devices.

To find out how many you have, count the items in your house that have a remote control, a continuous display or digital clock, an LED status light, or an external power adapter plug that looks like a big black cube with two prongs. Determine which items you can turn off while you are asleep or away from home. Plug several of them into the same power strip, and turn off the power strip to cut power to the devices.

If this isn't practical for you, consider the Smart Strip. This surge protector automatically cuts power to several energy leakers connected to it whenever you turn off the item plugged into its control outlet. For example, turning off a television plugged into the control outlet could also cut power to the cable box and DVD player. Although the Smart Strip costs around $30 at *www.amazon.com* or *www.smarthomeusa.com*, its makers claim you could save up to $240 a year after the Smart Strip pays for itself.

Cut your lighting bill with high-tech bulbs

Household lighting bills average at least $50 a year. You pay roughly $5 a year to power each incandescent bulb in your home, $3.50 for each halo gen bulb, and $1 for any CFL or LED bulb with the Energy Star label. CFL and LED bulbs give you the same level of brightness from fewer watts.

So check the bulb's label, and look for 450 lumens to replace a 40-watt bulb, 800 lumens for a 60-watt bulb, 1,100 lumens for a 75-watt bulb replacement, and 1,600 lumens for a 100-watt bulb. CFLs are usually the most cost effective, but LEDs are catching up as their prices drop.

Also check labels for recommended uses and to help compare costs. For example, LEDs recommended for outdoor fixtures may be better than CFLs because they come on instantly, last longer, and will not attract bugs.

Curb cooling costs with plants. South-facing or west-facing rooms can be blazing hot in the summer if no shade protects them from the sun. For ground floor rooms, rig up a tall string trellis from an old screen door or other found items, place the trellis so it can shade the window, and train one or two annual vines to climb it all summer long. You can even rig up a wider string trellis with more vines to protect the outside wall section for that room.

For second-story windows, plant the vines and a smaller trellis in a window box. Pull down the vines at the end of the growing season, so winter sun can warm these rooms.

Be prepared, not scared, when catastrophe strikes

"I never expected to wait a week before I could buy gas or groceries, cook food, or even refill my prescriptions," said Mary, after surviving a monster storm. "I couldn't even get to the documents we needed for insurance claims and emergency assistance."

Mary's experience shows why preparing early can help ease your stress considerably. When a disaster is fast approaching, you will not have enough time or opportunity to decide what you need and to buy all your supplies.

If the disaster occurs suddenly, roads may be impassable, power may be out, and stores may be closed. Even if a disaster is predicted several days in advance, roads often become clogged, and stores quickly run out of things you need. But if you have prepared long before a disaster, you have what you need, you know what to do, and you won't be as distressed or frightened. Start preparing with these ideas.

Plan a disaster kit. You don't need to prepare for every possible disaster. So once you have filled your disaster kit with standard supplies, only add supplies for the disasters likely in your area. Update the foods and medicines in your kit every six months, preferably on memorable holidays such as Memorial Day and Thanksgiving.

Be prepared with the basics. Start stocking your home so you're always ready for an emergency. Include these items:

- three-day supply of water (one gallon per person per day)
- three-day supply of nonperishable food. Stick with low-salt foods, or everyone will drink more.
- manual can opener
- flashlight
- matches in a waterproof container
- whistle
- battery-powered hand-crank radio
- spare batteries
- multipurpose tool
- one-week supply of medications and medical devices
- personal hygiene items, toilet paper, and sanitizing supplies
- garbage bags
- cell phone with charger
- family and emergency contact information
- extra cash
- emergency blankets
- disaster-specific supplies
- first aid kit

- copies of important personal, financial, medical, and legal documents

Older adults have a higher risk of dehydration, so add extra water for each person over age 50, and include canned foods with a high liquid content. Also, don't forget to plan for special dietary requirements such as sugar-free foods for people with diabetes or high-fiber foods to help prevent constipation.

Fill your first aid kit. Buy a prestocked kit, and add the following items if they are not already included.

- nonprescription antidiarrhea drugs and pain relievers
- thermometer
- hand sanitizer
- antiseptic wipes
- N95 surgical masks and medical-grade nonlatex gloves
- antibacterial ointment
- cotton balls
- adhesive tape and several types of nonstick bandages
- scissors, tweezers, and safety pins

Gather financial and household documents. To make filing insurance claims, receiving emergency assistance, and other tasks easier after a disaster, make three copies of:

- ownership documents like deeds, titles, receipts, and stock certificates.
- identifying documents such as social security cards, birth certificates, marriage certificates, military records, and driver's licenses.

- financial records like retirement account information, credit cards, proof of investments, and recent pay stubs, tax returns, and banking statements.

- insurance documents including insurance or Medicare cards.

- employee and government benefits information.

- household inventory.

Also include a list of items that may not appear on these documents like account numbers, insurance policy numbers, and customer service numbers for financial and insurance firms with whom you do business.

If you have not created a household inventory, visit *www.knowyourstuff.org* for a free smartphone application to help. To create your inventory without software, use a notebook and camera to record and describe every item in each room of your house. Include each item's cost, when you bought it, and how many you have. Pay special attention to valuables, but take pictures of everything. This pays off when you file insurance claims.

Include important health info. Make copies of the following information, and keep it in at least three places, including your wallet or purse and the places you store backup copies of financial documents.

- list of your doctors and their phone numbers

- list of the medications you take, the dosage, and how often you take them

- copies of prescriptions including your eyeglass prescription

- list of emergency contacts

- poison control and other emergency services telephone numbers

- allergies and immunization records

- list of your health conditions like diabetes or high blood pressure, plus important health facts such as having a pacemaker

For even better results, create a Personal Health Record (PHR) that includes this information and your medical history. Store it with your backup copies of other key documents. For a free PHR form you can print and fill out, visit *www.myphr.com*, or talk to your insurer. If possible, get copies of your medical and dental records to store with your backup copies of crucial documents.

To top off your medical preparations, add extra supplies to your disaster kit to help manage your specific ongoing health concerns such as arthritis pain, incontinence, or migraines.

Store paperwork in several places. Keep copies of your documents in at least two of these places — a lockable safe deposit box at home, a safe deposit box at your bank, or with a trusted out-of-town relative. Why? Documents at home are immediately available and can be evacuated with you. Documents at the bank will be there even if you "lose everything." Documents stored with an out-of-town relative can help after a region-wide disaster like a hurricane, when your bank safe deposit box may be unreachable for a long time.

Choose a few smart extras. These little gems can be priceless when you deal with a disaster or its aftermath.

- A small product called the SteriPen can quickly sterilize a quart of water as long as that water is clear and free of particles. The SteriPen costs around $60. It may be particularly useful if you can't store or carry enough jugs of water to last until water is available again or until you can return home after an evacuation.

- Dental floss is ideal for tying and securing things.

- Choose a few items for stress management such as nonperishable comfort foods, materials for writing and mailing letters to friends and relatives, a notebook to keep a journal of your experience, a Bible, or a few special photos.

- Include a notebook, pens, and a folder for documenting expenses and losses. Your written records, receipts, and any other paperwork should help when you talk with your insurance adjuster.

Disaster plan for disabilities

Talk to your doctor about what to add to your disaster kit if you or a loved one has a disability or chronic health condition. For example, you may need one or more of these:

- extra batteries for a hearing aid, electronic wheelchair, or diabetes meter

- medical ID bracelet

- names and serial numbers of your medical devices — including internal devices like a pacemaker

- backup power supply for your oxygen tank, scooter, or another medical device

- manual versions of wheelchairs or other medical equipment

- two-week supply of items you use daily or weekly for your health concern

Also, ask your doctor what other disaster preparations and plans you should make to accommodate the condition or disability.

6 smart ways to ease vacation health worries

You love taking vacations, but all those news stories about biting bedbugs, germy hotel rooms, and medical emergencies make you nervous. If you feel as if you just trade hometown stress for travel stress, start making plans to prevent or solve vacation health problems. Smart preparations like these can go a long way towards relieving your travel worries.

Keep an eye out for bedbugs. Bedbugs are making a comeback. They may not carry diseases, but they still bite humans to feed — and they keep coming back for more. That's why you never want to bring these little pests back from your vacation. Remember these four tips to help keep bedbugs out of your home.

- Inspect your hotel mattress the moment you arrive. Pull back the linens, and examine the mattress seams for black or reddish brown specks or bugs. Also, check the headboard and box springs. If you find signs of bedbugs, ask for a new room, and inspect it, too.

- Never place luggage on the carpet, bed, upholstered furniture, or any furniture near the bed in your hotel room. Instead, put the luggage on hard-surfaced furniture or on the tiled floor in the bathroom.

- When you return home, empty the clothes from your suitcase into plastic bags before entering the house. Even if you never wore these clothes, immediately wash them in hot water, and dry on high heat in the dryer for at least 20 minutes.

- Keep the empty luggage outside or in a sealed garbage can until you can store it for several hours in temperatures over 120 degrees. A car parked in the sun on a blazing hot day may reach 120 degrees as long as the windows are rolled up. If that's not an option, store the luggage where temperatures will stay below 22 degrees for two weeks.

If you suspect bedbugs have infested your home, think twice before using a bug fogger. A recent study suggests foggers may not kill most bedbugs because the bugs can hide in crevices the fog cannot reach. Experts recommend calling a professional exterminator to deal with bedbugs.

Stop traveler's constipation. A healthy salad made with delicious high-fiber foods can put an end to traveler's constipation before it starts. Numerous studies have found that fiber helps keep you regular. Try eating almonds, carrots, chickpeas, mushrooms, peppers, raisins, raspberries, and sunflower seeds every day during your vacation, and drink plenty of water. These tasty tactics may also help clear up any constipation you already have.

Fight back against fatigue. Need more energy and stamina to do all the things you want to do on vacation? If you feel tired all the time, you may want to try the Asian herb Siberian ginseng. One study found that four 500-milligram (mg) capsules a day helped reduce fatigue in people with mild chronic fatigue symptoms. But this herb may not be safe if you have certain health conditions, so talk to your doctor before you try it.

Prevent blisters. Friction causes blisters, but you can take steps to prevent it. Avoid friction from sweaty feet by using cornstarch, talcum powder, or commercial foot powder in your socks or shoes. You can also lubricate specific trouble spots — or your entire feet — with petroleum jelly.

Walk pain-free. All-day treks through amusement parks, shopping centers, or other tourist attractions can leave your legs sore, stiff, and maybe even weak. But don't let that spoil your vacation plans. Simple secrets like these could make all the difference.

- Chug some cherry juice. Research suggests you can expect less pain, less inflammation, and more rapid muscle recovery from intense exercise if you drink tart cherry juice every day. You should start at least four days before your first strenuous day and keep drinking the juice until at least two days after your last day of endless walking.

- Drink chocolate milk. Your muscles need to recover, repair, and rebuild themselves after intense exercise. Low-fat or nonfat chocolate milk may help. This yummy drink provides the proteins your muscles need to rebuild plus the carbohydrates that help refuel those muscles. Research suggests this helps prepare your muscles for the next round of walking. For best results, drink 8 to 16 ounces of chocolate milk within the first 30 minutes after you stop walking.

- Think ginkgo. Leg cramps or pain from walking may be a sign of peripheral artery disease (PAD) or intermittent claudication (IC), especially if the pain vanishes when you rest your legs. Only a doctor can tell whether you have PAD or a different problem, so check with your doctor to find out.

  Exercise therapy is a powerful way to fight the pain of IC and PAD, so you may want to try that first. But if you still have pain, one herb could hold the key — ginkgo biloba. PAD or IC pain is caused by poor circulation in your legs. But the leaf extract of ginkgo thins the blood and releases compounds like nitric oxide to help improve poor circulation.

In fact, studies suggest 120 mg of ginkgo in divided doses each day helps ease IC symptoms. It may be particularly effective when added to an exercise program. But ginkgo may not be safe to take with most medicines used to treat IC and PAD, so get your doctor's permission before you try this herb.

Avoid healthcare hassles on vacation. You already know which hometown hospital, doctor, and pharmacy to visit if you get sick or injured. But when you travel, that familiar safety net is gone. Build a vacation safety net to help you get better, safer, and less expensive treatment if you need it.

To begin, find out what your insurance policy covers when you travel. For example, medical evacuation or treatment at foreign hospitals may not be covered. If you find significant gaps in your policy, consider shopping around for temporary travel medical insurance.

But don't stop there. Find out which hospitals and pharmacies near your vacation destination are in your insurance network, and check the quality of the hospitals at the website *www.HospitalCompare.hhs.gov.*

Finally, don't forget to keep your insurance identification card and a list of your medications with you at all times during your vacation. If you have a chronic condition, also fill out the short medical history form available from the American College of Emergency Physicians at *www.emergencycarefor you.org/medicalforms.* Keep that form with your insurance card and medications list.

Prevent a painful suitcase surprise

In 2012, an injury caused by a suitcase forced Milwaukee Brewers baseball star Jonathan Lucroy off the field for several weeks. In fact, more than 54,000 Americans were treated for luggage-related injuries in one year alone. To prevent your suitcases from causing pains, strains, and stress, use these tips.

- Choose luggage with wheels and a handle. If new luggage is too expensive, consider a collapsible aluminum luggage cart to carry your bags.

- Make your luggage lighter. Choose sample-sized toiletries from stores like Sephora.com or Target, or buy empty containers marked "TSA-approved," and fill them with toiletries from home.

- Before placing a carry-on bag in the plane's overhead compartment, rest it on top of the seat, and grip it on the left and right sides. Lift the bag's wheels into the compartment first, and use one hand to push the bag fully inside.

Fly smart and safe

Flying the "friendly skies" may raise your risk of colds, blood clots, infections, and motion sickness, but simple precautions can help protect you. Before you buy a ticket, arm yourself with these secrets for a healthier, more relaxing trip.

Be spry in the sky. You don't have to line dance in the plane's aisle, but you should move around once an hour during the flight. This lowers your odds of deep vein thrombosis (DVT), the formation of a blood clot in your leg or pelvis. DVT can be fatal if the clot breaks away and blocks a blood vessel in your lungs. To prevent this, the American College of Chest Physicians (ACCP) suggests you walk or do calf exercises frequently during a flight, and drink plenty of water, especially on flights longer than six hours. People with above-normal risk should also reserve an aisle seat and wear graduated compression stockings. You may have a high risk of DVT if you:

- are an older adult or obese.

- have a history of DVT.

- have had recent surgery or a traumatic injury.

- have limited mobility.

- use estrogen or oral contraceptives.

- are confined in a window seat on the plane.

But be aware that the ACCP now recommends against taking aspirin to help prevent DVT. And, although DVT is often called "economy class syndrome," the ACCP has found that traveling in business class or first class does not lower your DVT risk.

Prevent colds on the fly. The air inside a plane is as dry as a desert, and viruses thrive there. What's more, the dry air cripples part of your defense system against viruses. To fight back, drink 8 ounces of caffeine-free, alcohol-free liquids each hour to prevent dehydration, and lubricate your nose with a saline nasal spray. If the saline spray usually fails to keep your poor nose from drying out, apply a tiny amount of saline nasal gel just inside the edges of your nostrils with a cotton swab before boarding the plane. You can find Ayr or another saline nasal gel near the saline nasal sprays in many stores.

Beware of germs on a plane. The plane's air is not the only place germs lurk. In fact, many kinds of dangerous germs may be waiting for you on clean-looking surfaces inside the cabin. Remember, viruses can live for up to one day on some surfaces, so the germs may linger after a previous passenger has gone.

Seat-back pockets, tray tables, airline blankets and pillows, and the airplane's bathroom are notorious germ carriers, so plan accordingly. Carry your own reading material, and avoid the seat-back pocket completely. Bring a disinfecting wipe to clean the tray table before you use it, and wipe down the seat armrests and seat belt buckle, too. Never use the airline's blankets or pillows. Instead, dress in extra layers to keep warm, and bring your own travel pillow.

Use a paper towel to close the toilet lid in the plane's bathroom before flushing, and be sure to "wash" your hands with a 70-percent alcohol hand sanitizer before returning to your seat. In fact, use hand sanitizer often while on the plane and in the airport. In addition to germy spots on planes, security checkpoints, baggage areas, and check-in kiosks also harbor germs.

Avoid motion sickness. Use these tips to start preventing motion sickness long before you set eyes on your plane.

- Book a seat by the wings so you feel less movement.

- Take a medicine to prevent motion sickness 30 minutes before you board. Choices include over-the-counter options like dimenhydrinate (Dramamine), meclizine (Bonine) or a longer-lasting prescription patch.

- Don't board with an empty stomach. One study found that people were more likely to get motion sickness if they had eaten nothing than if they had drunk a protein shake first.

- Bring glossy magazines to stack in your seat. Some people report that sitting on a slippery surface or stack of magazines helps keep motion sickness at bay. The work your brain must do to keep you balanced on that slippery surface may be enough to interfere with the processes that cause motion sickness.

Free TSA hotline for travelers with medical needs

Making your way through the airport security checkpoint can be a major hurdle if you have special medical needs or a disability. Fortunately, the TSA now offers a toll-free number where you can get help.

Call TSA Cares toll-free at 855-787-2227 for information about what you can expect at the security checkpoint based on your medical conditions and disabilities. You can also ask questions about screening procedures and policies.

A TSA representative will address your concerns about items like a CPAP machine, walker, orthopedic shoes, oxygen supply, diabetes testing meter, implanted device, prosthetic or brace, your service dog, or any disability. Call between 9 a.m. and 9 p.m. Eastern time on a weekday, but be sure to call at least three business days before you plan to travel.

Super strategies to live long and strong

Tasty ways to fight Alzheimer's disease

You don't need exotic fruits and expensive juices to guard your brain into old age. Science shows some of your favorite, everyday foods offer potent protection against mental decline and dementia.

Crack open a can. Salmon is a top source of DHA and EPA, two types of omega-3 fatty acids. New evidence shows they can protect your brain from the ravages of aging.

More than 1,500 seniors underwent blood tests measuring their omega-3 levels, MRI scans, and exams to test their memory and thinking skills. Those with the lowest omega-3 in their blood scored the worst on tests of visual memory, problem solving, abstract thinking, and multi-tasking.

"People with lower blood levels of omega-3 fatty acids had lower brain volumes that were equivalent to about two years of structural brain aging," explains Zaldy Tan, with the Easton

Center for Alzheimer's Disease Research at the University of California, Los Angeles. Past research has shown that people with the highest DHA levels enjoyed a 37-percent lower risk of Alzheimer's disease (AD) and a 47-percent lower risk of dementia from all causes.

Experts say you get most of your omega-3 from eating fish. Fresh fish isn't always cheap, but canned salmon can deliver these nutrients at a price that's right.

Bite into an apple. A fruit straight out of the Bible may help protect you from Alzheimer's disease. Mice with AD had improved brain function after drinking the equivalent of two to three 8-ounce glasses of apple juice each day for a month.

Apple juice reduced the buildup of damaging free radicals in their brains, but it may also boost acetylcholine, a chemical that helps brain cells communicate, improving memory. In fact, research suggests you could noticeably improve your memory just by eating a couple of these juicy fruits. Getting the human equivalent of two glasses of apple juice or two to three apples daily boosted acetylcholine levels, memory, and mental function in mice.

Apples and apple juice are rich in protective antioxidants. These potent compounds prevent the drop in brain levels of acetylcholine that comes with age. That's important, because a fall in acetylcholine has been linked to Alzheimer's disease, along with memory problems and poorer brain function.

Science shows the nutrients in apples could also aid weight loss and help fight a slew of other illnesses, including:

- heart disease.
- lung cancer.
- breast cancer.

- colon cancer.

- type 2 diabetes.

- damage to your stomach lining caused by nonsteroidal anti-inflammatory drugs like ibuprofen.

- stomach cancer.

Shop for cloudy apple juice and fresh juice made from cider apples. These pack more healthy antioxidants than clear juice and juice made from dessert apples.

Eat to beat Alzheimer's

Take a look at these 12 fabulous foods. Each is packed with nutrients and other compounds that may protect your memories from the ravages of Alzheimer's disease.

- canned salmon for omega-3

- eggs for choline

- fortified breakfast cereals for niacin

- frozen berries for antioxidants

- apples for antioxidants

- nuts for vitamin E, monounsaturated fat, and polyunsaturated fat

- Brussels sprouts for vitamin C

- spinach for folate

- rosemary for antioxidants and aromatherapy

- coffee for caffeine

- tea for L-theanine

- milk for vitamin D

Go nuts, in a good way. A strong study out of New York suggests you could shield your brain from Alzheimer's just by eating the right combination of foods. One of them — nuts, for their rich stores of vitamin E.

More than 2,000 New York seniors told researchers what they typically ate, then underwent tests for dementia every year and a half. Those who ate a diet rich in nuts, fish, tomatoes, poultry, and fruits, along with cruciferous, dark, and green leafy vegetables were nearly 40 percent less likely to develop Alzheimer's.

Besides vitamin E, nuts are top-notch sources of healthy unsaturated fats. These may protect your brain by preventing hardening of the arteries, blood clots, and inflammation, plus block the buildup of beta-amyloid in your brain.

- For vitamin E, choose almonds, hazelnuts, and peanuts.

- For monounsaturated fat, you can't beat macadamia nuts, hazelnuts, and pecans.

- For polyunsaturated fat, take your pick of walnuts, pecans, and peanuts.

Stock up on spinach. The same New York study that recognized nuts for fighting AD also linked leafy greens like spinach to a lower risk of this disease. Spinach is chock-full of folate, a B vitamin that reduces the amount of homocysteine in your blood. High levels of this amino acid are linked to higher risk of Alzheimer's disease and a drop in brain performance. For each tiny, 1-micromole increase in your homocysteine, your risk of AD rises 16 percent. One recent study showed that seniors who got the most folate daily were half as likely to develop AD.

Experts say the evidence isn't strong enough to recommend supplements, but foods are always a safe bet. Put the odds in your favor by loading up on spinach and other sources of folate. Leafy green vegetables, lentils, pinto beans, black beans, and many fortified breakfast cereals provide plenty.

Be choosy about B12

Vitamin B12 may also protect you from Alzheimer's disease (AD). It's found in plenty of foods, but be warned — some of them may do your brain more harm than good.

In one study, however, people with the lowest risk of AD actually got the least B12. That's because many foods rich in B12, like meat and dairy, are also high in saturated fat. That, in turn, may increase your odds of getting this disease.

Instead, look for low-fat food sources like fish; poultry; and low-fat and fat-free milk, yogurt, and cottage cheese. Supplements can help some people but not everyone. Your stomach must produce a substance called intrinsic factor to absorb B12, and it may not produce enough as you get older. Without it, you'll need B12 injections.

Your doctor can spot a B12 deficiency with a simple blood test, then help you decide the best way to boost your levels.

Break out the Brussels sprouts. These cruciferous vegetables are bursting with vitamin C, a nutrient that may reduce your risk of Alzheimer's. Some research suggests that getting enough vitamin C from food, along with vitamin E, may help prevent this deadly disease.

It's the most efficient of all the antioxidants. Antioxidants scavenge molecules called free radicals that damage the DNA inside your cells. Your body also needs antioxidants to repair that DNA. Free radical damage is key in the development of Alzheimer's. It can kill brain cells and contributes to the brain changes that mark AD.

Vitamin C neutralizes these dangerous compounds better than vitamin E or any other nutrient. And with nearly 100 milligrams (mg) of vitamin C per cup, Brussels sprouts are one of the best sources. Strawberries, orange juice, sweet red and green peppers, and broccoli are no slouches, either.

Experts say eating plenty of fruits and vegetables, along with taking a supplement — as little as 30 or 60 mg of vitamin C daily — can ensure you get enough to guard your brain.

Add a dash of rosemary. This fragrant herb may give your memory a lift. The ancient Greek physician Pedanius Dioscorides wrote of rosemary, "The eating of its flower in a preserve comforts the brain, ... sharpens understanding, restores lost memory, awakens the mind."

Modern science seems to agree. Researchers gave 28 seniors different doses of dried rosemary, then tested their memory skills for several hours afterward. Surprisingly, the lowest dose of rosemary — closest to the amount you would use in cooking — had the biggest impact. This small amount sped up memory recall, a potential predictor of brain function. Rosemary is teeming with antioxidants that may protect your brain. Its compounds may keep acetylcholine from breaking down.

Simply smelling this herb may boost your brain. People who sniffed rosemary essential oil in a recent study scored better on tests of brain performance, especially on speed and accuracy. The scent even improved their mood.

The smell seems to help people with Alzheimer's disease, too. Japanese researchers placed oils in diffusers — aromatherapy gadgets with a small fan — in rooms with elderly people who had dementia.

- In the morning, the seniors smelled a mixture of rosemary and lemon essential oils. This combination boosts concentration and memory.

- In the evening, people switched to smelling lavender and orange essential oils, to calm them.

It worked. After four weeks, researchers tested the seniors and found they had become better at understanding concepts and abstract ideas — even the seniors with Alzheimer's disease. Start incorporating rosemary into your everyday recipes, and take a deep breath of it while you cook. You may do your brain a favor.

Build a breakfast that feeds your brain

Some traditional breakfast items are proven brain-boosters. They're packed with nutrients that ward off memory loss, mental decline, and even dementia. Pair these foods together for a morning meal that really gets you going.

Pour a cup of protection. Coffee just keeps getting better. This super drink packs more soluble fiber than orange juice, and now experts think it may ward off the mental decline of Alzheimer's.

Each year, 15 percent of seniors with mild cognitive impairment (MCI) progress to full-blown Alzheimer's disease. Experts wondered why some people with MCI develop AD while others don't. So they tested a group of seniors with MCI.

Those who ended up with Alzheimer's over the next two to four years had half as much caffeine in their blood as those who didn't get the disease. The cutoff between those who did get AD and those who didn't was about the same as drinking several cups of coffee over a few hours.

"Moderate daily consumption of caffeinated coffee appears to be the best dietary option for long-term protection against Alzheimer's memory loss," according to Gary Arendash, recently retired Research Professor of Cell Biology, Microbiology, and Molecular Biology at the University of South Florida (USF). "Coffee is inexpensive, readily available, easily gets into the brain, and has few side effects for most of us. Moreover, our studies show that caffeine and coffee appear to directly attack the Alzheimer's disease process."

"These intriguing results suggest that older adults with mild memory impairment who drink moderate levels of coffee — about three cups a day — will not convert to Alzheimer's disease, or at least will experience a substantial delay before converting to Alzheimer's," adds Chuanhai Cao, a neuroscientist at the USF Health Byrd Alzheimer's Institute.

Add to that the science suggesting coffee helps protect you from diabetes, skin cancer, heart disease, breast cancer, Parkinson's disease, and lethal prostate cancer, and you can feel better about your java-drinking habit.

10 foods you shouldn't do without

They're some of the healthiest and most inexpensive foods you can buy. Some you can even grow yourself. And all of them are proven to guard your brain against mental decline and dementia.

- apples
- coffee
- spinach
- canned salmon
- milk

- frozen berries
- tea
- Brussels sprouts
- fortified breakfast cereal
- eggs

Brew a brain cocktail. Not a coffee drinker? Never fear. Tea can give you a fast mental boost, too. Its combination of caffeine and L-theanine, an amino acid, seems to speed up thinking and improve concentration.

People who drink tea throughout the day may perceive things faster. That's what happened in one study when people were given small amounts of caffeine throughout the day — the same amount as in a cup of tea.

In fact, the brain-boosting benefits of tea may even outclass coffee. Tea may ramp up your perception faster and maintain it longer. Experts think the L-theanine:

- improves concentration by revving up alpha-wave activity in your brain. Alpha activity is linked to better learning and concentration, and better performance under stress.

- enhances the positive effects of caffeine, speeding up your reaction time, helping your brain process information faster, reducing tiredness and mental fatigue, and making you more alert.

These benefits could start with as little as two cups of tea. You may be fighting AD, too, thanks to antioxidants in both green and black teas. The epigallocatechin gallate in green tea and theaflavins in black tea may stop the development of toxic amyloid proteins linked to Alzheimer's and Parkinson's diseases.

Munch for better memories. Cereal isn't just for kids. Eating one fortified with niacin could help you dodge dementia down the road. This B vitamin:

- helps turn glucose into energy.

- raises your "good" HDL cholesterol as much as 35 percent.

- lowers "bad" LDL cholesterol as much as 20 percent.

- may protect against Alzheimer's and declining brain function with age.

Niacin deficiency can cause dementia and confusion, but even a low-grade shortage has an impact. Researchers found that people in Chicago who routinely got the least niacin from food saw a bigger drop in brain function over five and a half years. They were also more likely to develop AD.

This B vitamin plays a major role in building and repairing DNA, growing the connections between brain cells, and guarding your brain from free radical damage.

Fortunately, it's easy to find. A single cup of General Mill's Total Raisin Bran delivers 21 mg of niacin, nearly twice what the government says you need each day. Other fortified cereals are close behind.

Do your body good. Adding milk to your cereal makes it even better brain food. That's because dairy is a solid source of vitamin D. A 2009 study found that people who weren't getting enough vitamin D had double the risk of memory loss and cognitive impairment. In a new study, the same researchers discovered that seniors who were the most vitamin D deficient were four times more likely to develop cognitive impairment.

This nutrient plays many roles in your body. You know what it does for your bones, but did you know it helps clear toxic beta-amyloid protein from your brain? Or that it protects your brain from free radical damage? It even influences the growth and development of nerve tissue. That helps explain why a shortage increases your risk for neurological diseases, like Parkinson's disease and multiple sclerosis. Getting too little vitamin D may also raise your risk of type 2 diabetes, which in turn could lead to cognitive impairment.

The recommended amount is 600 international units (IU) for people under age 70 and 800 IU for those over age 70. Protect your brain and your precious memories. Make low-fat and nonfat milk, yogurt, and other dairy part of your daily routine. Your doctor can measure your vitamin D levels with a simple blood test.

How savvy shoppers save on milk

Stock up on milk when it goes on sale. Look for jugs with the furthest expiration date. Then bring the milk home and freeze it for future use.

- First, pour out a glass to drink. Like other liquids, milk expands when it freezes. This empties enough from the jug to keep it from exploding in the freezer.

- Replace the cap tightly, pop it in the icebox, and store for up to one month.

- Thaw it by setting the jug in a sink of water overnight.

- Shake it thoroughly the next morning and pour. Refrigerate as usual.

Bring on the berries. Sprinkle a handful of blueberries, straw-berries, or raspberries on your cereal every morning to keep your memory sharp. Researchers analyzed all of the studies done on berries and the brain. Strong evidence shows they boost brain function and help prevent age-related memory loss.

- Berries are chock-full of antioxidants, compounds that protect your brain cells from damage by free radicals.

- Berries change how brain cells communicate with each other. These signaling changes can prevent inflammation that would otherwise harm brain cells.

- By preventing inflammation, they also improve thinking ability and muscle control.

A separate study found that berries such as blueberries, straw-berries, and acai may trigger your brain's housekeeping mechanism, prompting cells called microglia to sweep away debris that can interfere with brain function. Microglia stop working as you age, but berries may help reverse that.

Don't wait until they're in season. Frozen berries make afford-able, year-round treats. Buy them at your favorite grocery store or freeze your own from your garden.

Unscramble your memory. New research suggests the choline you get from eggs and other foods could improve your mem-ory and maybe even ward off age-related mental decline and dementias such as Alzheimer's disease.

Your body needs this essential nutrient to make acetylcholine, a chemical that enables brain cells to talk to each other. It's crucial for memory. Having enough choline in your brain may preserve brain cells and the pathways to verbal and visual memory. Protecting these paths is key to preventing the brain changes that lead to Alzheimer's disease.

Women over the age of 51 need at least 425 milligrams (mg) of choline each day — men need 550 mg. Eggs get you off to a great start. A breakfast of two large eggs meets half your daily needs with 232 mg of choline. Milk and peanuts are other good sources.

Surprising ways to manage chronic pain

"Pain, pain go away. Come again some other day." If only it were as easy as singing a rhyme, you would have banished your aches long ago. Don't give up — pain doesn't have to be a part of your life.

Turn to an herb. Lower back pain affecting your life? Try a little-known herbal remedy. It goes by the unfortunate name "devil's claw," but it could be a blessing in disguise. Research suggests it may relieve lower back pain as well as a powerful prescription pain medicine.

Look for a supplement that will give you at least 50 milligrams (mg) of harpagoside a day, the herb's active painkilling ingredient. While it seems to be safe, you should:

- avoid it if you have ulcers or you take a blood thinner such as warfarin (Coumadin), since the combination could increase your risk of bleeding.

- stop taking it two weeks before surgery or any procedure that carries a chance of bleeding, and wait awhile before you begin it again.

Fish for relief. Ibuprofen, naproxen, and other nonsteroidal anti-inflammatories (NSAIDs) aren't suited for everyone because of their side effects. Up to half of people who take them develop dyspepsia. Two out of 10 get ulcers. Almost everyone develops stomach bleeding with long-term use.

Fish oil may offer a safer but equally effective alternative. Doctors already know this natural supplement can help relieve arthritis pain, but evidence suggests it may relieve back and neck pain, too.

Two neurologists grew tired of giving their patients NSAIDs for pain, so they investigated fish oil supplements.

- For the first two weeks, they gave 250 people with neck and back pain 2.4 grams (g) of pharmaceutical-grade fish oil, in addition to their regular NSAIDs.

- After two weeks, the doctors began tapering off the NSAID medications. They also cut back the fish oil dosage to 1.2 g each day.

- Less than three months later, six out of every 10 people had given up their pain pills.

These experts think two out of three people taking NSAIDs could come off them with the help of fish oil supplements. Side effects are rare, but avoid fish oil if you take blood-thinning medications or are allergic to fish.

Adjust your attitude. Focus less on your pain, and you'll sleep better and hurt less.

"We have found that people who ruminate about their pain and have more negative thoughts about their pain don't sleep as well, and the result is they feel more pain," says Luis F. Buenaver, assistant professor of psychiatry and behavioral sciences at Johns Hopkins University School of Medicine. "It may sound simple," he adds, "but you can change the way you feel by changing the way you think."

Research shows that negative thinking makes you sleep worse, and poor sleep makes you more sensitive to pain. Believe it or not, changing the way you think may ease your pain just as much as sleeping pills and painkillers.

A special type of treatment known as cognitive behavioral therapy (CBT) can help you head off negative thoughts. It's been proven to treat pain from temporomandibular joint disorder, but it may also aid fibromyalgia, irritable bowel syndrome, neck and back pain, and certain types of headaches. Look for a psychologist, psychiatrist, or social worker specially trained in CBT.

Sleep it off. It can be hard to sleep deeply when you hurt, but sleeping badly or not enough magnifies pain. That's why it's important to do everything you can to get a good night's rest.

Poor sleep boosts inflammation. Inflammation, in turn, worsens pain. Young women who had their nightly sleep cut in half, from eight to four hours, for 10 days not only experienced a rise in inflammatory compounds in their blood — they also reported hurting worse during the day.

Getting a good night's rest can quench inflammation. And that could ease chronic pain. Try this advice for deeper sleep.

- Dim the lights inside your home before bedtime to trigger your body to make melatonin.

- Don't watch TV before bed. It's too stimulating. Do something crafty with your hands, instead. This will soothe your mind into a peaceful state.

- Place a cool, damp washcloth on your forehead at night to fight insomnia and help you drift off faster, or tuck an ice pack in your pillow case. Cool temperatures quiet part of the brain linked to insomnia.

For more advice on getting a good night's sleep, head to the *Best ways to beat fatigue and boost energy* chapter.

Play your favorite music. If you tend to get swept up easily in a good book or other activity, then music may relieve your pain.

Listening to music distracted people from their pain when they were shocked on the fingertip. Researchers told them to focus on the music, follow the melody, and try to pick out unusual tones in it.

Music activates pathways in your brain and body that compete with pain for your attention. Activities that occupy your brain also cause it to release opioids. These chemicals block pain signals from moving up your spinal cord and reaching your brain. The more anxious you are, the more music may help.

So the next time your back acts up or you visit the dentist, pop in some earphones and focus on your favorite tunes.

When vitamins kill

More of a good thing isn't always better. Megadoses of certain vitamins could increase your risk of disease, or even death.

Vitamin E. Experts once thought vitamin E supplements could ward off cancer. New research shows just the opposite. They actually raised men's risk of prostate cancer by 17 percent. "For the typical man, there appears to be no benefit in taking vitamin E, and in fact, there may be some harm," warns Eric Klein, chair of the Glickman Urological and Kidney Institute at Cleveland Clinic.

Another study found that large doses of E could increase your odds of dying. The risk began at 150 International Units (IU) of E each day, with real danger striking at 400 IU a day. That's big news. Half of people over age 60 take supplements containing vitamin E. One in four gets at least 400 IU daily.

Vitamin D. Too much vitamin D leads to dangerously high levels of calcium in your blood, damaging your bones, kidneys, and soft tissue. People who overdo it are almost always taking prescription vitamin D, not over-the-counter supplements. Published reports of vitamin D toxicity all involve taking at least 40,000 IU a day (1,000 micrograms). You cannot get toxic amounts of D from sunlight.

Vitamin A. The maximum amount of vitamin A that experts deem safe is 10,000 IU daily. But amounts ranging from 5,000 to 10,000 IU could put you in danger of developing osteoporosis and fracturing your hip. That's not all. Taking vitamin A in the form of retinyl palmitate or retinyl acetate has been linked to lung cancer, while high doses of A may raise your risk of dying.

Get focused. Training your brain through a process called "focused attention" could slash your pain in half. It even worked better than morphine in a new study.

- Start by sitting up straight with your eyes closed.

- Focus on your breathing. Pay attention to how the air feels going in and out of your nostrils.

- Shift your focus to the rise and fall of your chest and abdomen as you breathe in and out.

- Don't get frustrated if your mind gets sidetracked. Just return your attention to your breathing.

It's as easy as that. Fifteen people learned to do it in just four days. They spent 20 minutes practicing each day. Then researchers gave them painful jolts of heat while scanning their brains to see how they reacted. During the first heat test, participants were told to lie still with their eyes closed. During the second heat test, they were told to practice their new "focused attention" exercise.

The exercise changed the way people's brains processed pain signals. Among other things, it completely quieted the part of the brain that tells you where and how much something hurts.

People said the pain felt only half as unpleasant during the exercise as when they weren't practicing, and it felt much less intense.

"We found a big effect — about a 40-percent reduction in pain intensity and a 57-percent reduction in pain unpleasantness," says Fadel Zeidan, postdoctoral research fellow at Wake Forest Baptist Medical Center. Focused attention "produced a greater reduction in pain than even morphine or other pain-relieving drugs, which typically reduce pain ratings by about 25 percent."

These folks reaped results in as few as four days. Other studies suggest the more you practice, the more relief you may get.

Amazing natural cure for infections

What stops drug-resistant bacteria even better than antibiotics? Believe it or not, it's honey. This natural wonder can cure stubborn, chronic infections — as long as you use the right kind.

A recent test tube study found that methicillin-resistant staphylococcus aureus (MRSA) treated with manuka honey loses a protein it needs to survive. In fact, manuka honey successfully treated MRSA-infected wounds that antibiotics had failed to cure, one study reported. Another study discovered that manuka honey defeated MRSA in most chronic leg ulcers.

Laboratory research suggests manuka honey may kill other bacteria besides MRSA that form antibiotic resistant barriers, such as *pseudomonas aeruginosa*, *klebsiella pneumoniae*, and *streptococcus pyogenes*. But manuka honey can't cure every antibiotic-resistant problem, so see your doctor before you try to treat an infection yourself.

8 tricks to cut your risk of falling

Falling is the second most-common fatal accident. But it doesn't have to be. Protect yourself with a few simple tips.

Pop a piece of gum. The next time you find yourself standing in a long line, try chewing gum. Smacking on a stick may help you keep your balance when you stand still for long periods of time. In one study, people who chewed gum while standing were more stable and swayed less, even with their eyes closed.

Slip-proof your shoes. Nonslip treads aren't just for the bathtub. They may be a cheap way to keep from falling. Stick them to the inside of your shoes, on the insole, to stop your feet from sliding around. New research showed that shoes with textured insoles improved people's balance and kept them from swaying during tough balance tests.

Pour a glass of milk. Getting an adequate daily dose of vitamin D can bolster bones, strengthen muscles, curb your risk of certain cancers, including colon cancer, and help thwart arthritis.

Too little does just the opposite. "Low levels of vitamin D can contribute to a number of serious, potentially life-threatening conditions such as softened bones; diseases that cause progressive muscle weakness leading to an increased risk of falls; osteoporosis; cardiovascular disease; certain types of cancer; and type 2 diabetes," according to Robin Daly, Chair of Exercise and Aging in the Center for Physical Activity and Nutrition Research at Deakin University in Australia.

Vitamin D deficiency is a problem even in countries like Australia that get lots of sunshine. Daly's newest study found that nearly one-third of Australians are vitamin D deficient, including more than half of women over age 75.

Dairy can help fill the void. Outside of sunshine, it's one of the best sources of vitamin D. Plus, it won't give you a sunburn. An 8-ounce glass of low-fat milk delivers one-third of the vitamin D you need each day.

Milk on its own merits is good for you, too. Men who drank milk or otherwise ate dairy at least once a day were a whopping 65 percent less likely to become disabled or lose their ability to do normal, everyday activities.

Play a game. Grab a friend or spouse for a game of balloon volleyball or catch with a tennis ball. Low-impact activities like these sharpen the coordination between your body and your brain.

Add safety updates. No longer steady on your feet? You don't have to give up your independence just yet. A few cheap and easy changes around your house will help you live on your own longer and reduce your risk of falling. These eight essential safety products are missing from most people's homes. Do you have them?

- night lights between your bedroom and bathroom, and at the top and bottom of stairs

- raised toilet seats to make it easier to sit down and stand up

- grab bars inside the shower or tub and next to the toilet

- nonslip mats placed under rugs, or double-sided tape securing rugs to the floor

- 60- to 75-watt light bulbs in every room and stairway

- an easy-to-find flashlight on each level of your home, including one by the bed

- nonslip bath mats inside tubs and showers, or nonslip adhesive strips

- motion-activated lights in places you often enter with your hands full, such as the utility room and basement

Invest in hearing aids. Believe it or not, hearing loss affects your sense of balance. Older women with the worst hearing in one study were three to four times more likely to fall.

"Gait and balance are things most people take for granted, but they are actually very cognitively demanding," says Frank Lin, assistant professor at Johns Hopkins School of Medicine and Bloomberg School of Public Health. Your brain has to work extra hard to make up for poor hearing. That means it has less energy to devote to maintaining your balance.

Have your hearing checked by a doctor or audiologist. Get fitted for hearing aids if you need them, and have a professional show you how to adjust them properly. Be sure to wear one in each ear if you need it, for the best balance.

Try tai chi. This ancient Chinese art is enjoying a revival, as seniors and scientists alike realize its health benefits. Tai chi involves slow, gentle movements that anyone can do. Studies show it builds strength in your legs.

In fact, new research found that tai chi, not physical therapy, reduced the number of falls seniors took. Perhaps more importantly, tai chi classes made seniors more confident of their balance. Researchers think this new confidence made them less likely to fall.

Heartburn drugs put hips at risk

A particular type of heartburn medicine known as proton pump inhibitors (PPIs) makes you more likely to fracture a hip. And the longer you take them, the higher your risk.

Popular PPI drugs include omeprazole (Prilosec), esomeprazole (Nexium), lansoprazole (Prevacid), rabeprazole (Aciphex), pantoprazole (Protonix), and dexlansoprazole (Kapidex).

Postmenopausal women on a PPI for at least two years were 35 percent more likely to fracture a hip, particularly if they smoked. After six to eight years on the drug, that risk rose to 55 percent.

Experts aren't entirely sure why. These medicines may keep your body from absorbing calcium, interfere with bone growth, or lower bone mineral density by disrupting your thyroid gland.

Two years after they stopped taking the drug, women's risk of hip fracture had dropped to normal. Don't stop taking a PPI on your own, however. They are important medications. Consult your doctor and decide what's best together.

Tread carefully with these drugs. Common medications can trip you up. Those that depress your central nervous system, such as antidepressants and painkillers, slow down your reactions and make you less alert. That puts you at risk for falls. The worst offenders include:

- anticholinergics, such as chlordiazepoxide (Librium, Limbitrol).

- antidepressants, like sertraline, citalopram (Celexa), escitalopram (Lexapro), and fluoxetine (Prozac).

- antipsychotics, including risperidone (Risperdal), olanzapine (Zyprexa), and quetiapine (Seroquel).

- benzodiazepines, such as alprazolam (Xanax) and Valium.

- dopaminergic drugs used to treat Parkinson's disease.

- diuretics, especially hydrochlorothiazide (HydroDIURIL, among others) and furosemide (Lasix).

- sleep aids such as zolpidem (Ambien).

- anti-arrhythmia drugs, including digoxin (Cardoxin, others), procainamide (Procanbid), and quinidine.

The more medicines you take, the more likely you are to fall, too. "Falls are the leading cause of both fatal and nonfatal injuries for adults 65 and older, and research suggests that those taking four or more medications are at an even greater risk that those who don't — perhaps two to three times greater," says Susan Blalock, associate professor at the University of North Carolina Eshelman School of Pharmacy.

Prescription drugs aren't the only danger, however. Over-the-counter medicines can also raise your risk. "Some allergy medications, sleep aids, and some cold and cough remedies can have the same effects as prescription drugs," says Stefanie Ferreri, clinical assistant professor at the Eshelman School of Pharmacy.

Don't stop taking any of your medicines, even if you suspect they're affecting your balance. Instead, call your doctor or pharmacist, describe your concerns, and ask if there's a similar, safer drug you can take.

Simple ways to stay sharp and independent

Keep your body and mind in shape into your 90s — or even into your 100s. From feeling stronger and having more energy to thinking quicker and dodging dementia, these eight tips can keep you in tiptop physical and mental condition.

Chat with a friend. Striking up a conversation with someone while waiting in line could enhance your brain function. "Simply talking to other people, the way you do when you're making friends, can provide mental benefits," says psychologist Oscar Ybarra of the University of Michigan Institute for Social Research.

A friendly conversation where two people get to know each other can strengthen your problem-solving skills. Talking to someone in a combative way, on the other hand, won't.

"We believe that performance boosts come about because some social interactions induce people to try to read others' minds and take their perspectives on things," Ybarra explains.

Ybarra and his colleagues had people spend 10 minutes getting to know a perfect stranger, then tested their mental performance. This simple exercise gave a bump to executive function, the part of your mind that involves working memory and your ability to ignore distractions. It's crucial to handling life's everyday problems. In fact, past research shows social interactions give your brain a lift similar to doing brain games like crossword puzzles. So call up a friend and schedule a coffee date. You'll both benefit.

Consider a supplement. The substance carnitine helps your cells produce energy. It does most of its work in your heart and skeletal muscles. After you turn 70, the amount of carnitine in your body starts to drop. That's one reason seniors tend to lose muscle as they get older. Bumping up your levels may help maximize your energy.

- Thirty-two people over the age of 100 tried carnitine supplements in one recent study. They took 2 grams daily in a form known as levocarnitine (L-carnitine). Another 34 people received fake supplements, or placebos.

- After six months, those on carnitine had less body fat, more muscle, more energy, and better thinking skills. They were even able to walk farther.

L-carnitine supplements seem to be safe, except in people with seizure disorders. Always discuss supplements with your doctor before trying anything on your own, however. And don't buy D-carnitine by mistake. Only the L- version is active in your body.

Learn almost anything — for free

Go back to school from the comfort of your couch. Study art history, astronomy, even computer science. All you need is a computer or smartphone and a connection to the Internet.

High-quality websites created by universities and nonprofit organizations offer classes, lectures, and interviews with experts for free. Try these for starters.

- Academic Earth offers lectures by professors at some of the nation's best schools, including Harvard, M.I.T., Stanford, and Yale at *www.academicearth.org.*

- The Khan Academy can help you master your math skills or brush up on finance, all at your own pace at *www.khanacademy.org.*

- Coursera has partnered with some of the world's best universities to offer online college courses free through *www.coursera.org.*

- iTunes U boasts hundreds of thousands of videos and lectures from colleges and cultural institutions. Download the iTunes U app to your iPhone, iPod Touch, or iPad from *www.apple.com/education/itunes-u.*

Grab a good book. Reading and writing now may preserve your mind as you age. More than 1,000 seniors, average age of 80, underwent annual memory exams for around five years. Each time, they also told researchers how often they read the newspaper; wrote letters; visited the library; or played chess, checkers, or other board games.

Astonishingly, researchers could predict how well each person's mind would function at their next exam solely by looking at how often they did any of those activities the year before. "The results suggest a cause and effect relationship: that being mentally active leads to better cognitive health in old age," says Robert Wilson of Rush University Medical Center.

Challenging your brain with activities like reading and playing checkers actually changes your gray and white matter. These mental activities strengthen the cells and connections involved in thinking, the same way exercising a muscle makes it stronger.

Use the opposite hand. Something as simple as brushing your teeth with your opposite hand can strengthen your brain. Changing your routines exercises different, seldom-used pathways in your brain, keeping cells younger and stronger.

Of course, not every little change works your brain enough to make a difference. For instance, writing in pencil instead of writing in pen won't help any. It's not a big enough change. Writing with the opposite hand will. Or, if you use a computer, try moving your mouse with the opposite hand.

Exercises like these are called neurobics. To work, they must involve at least one of your senses (taste, touch, sight, smell, sound), keep your attention engaged, and switch up your routine in a surprising way. Try one of these "workouts" tomorrow.

- Get dressed with your eyes closed. It exercises your senses of touch and hearing in a new way.

- Brush your teeth with the opposite hand.

- Drive to the store by taking a route you've never gone before.

- Fish your keys out of your purse and unlock the door with your eyes closed the next time you return home.

Talk to yourself. The next time you get caught muttering to yourself in the grocery aisle, don't be embarrassed. A new study shows that talking to yourself gives you a brief mental boost.

Hearing the name of something you're looking for helps the visual system in your brain find the item faster. The next time you lose your keys, glasses, or cup of coffee, try repeating its name as you search the house. You just may find it more easily.

Take care of your teeth. The bacteria in your mouth could cause your hip or knee implant to fail. New evidence suggests the bacteria behind gum disease can sneak into your bloodstream and infect the fluid around these joints. Experts think these bad bugs may be one reason artificial joints sometimes fail in the first 10 years.

"For a long time, we've suspected that these bacteria were causing problems in arthritis patients, but never had the scientific evidence to support it," according to Nabil Bissada, chair of the Department of Periodontics at the Case Western Reserve University School of Dental Medicine.

Dr. Bissada's latest study looked at 36 people with gum disease, testing the fluid in their joints for signs of mouth bacteria. Eight had an artificial joint that failed. Of those, three had mouth bacteria in their joints.

When plaque bacteria break through the protective pocket surrounding your teeth, they can slip into the bloodstream. There, they hitch a ride to other parts of your body, stirring up inflammation. The problem has also been linked to heart disease, kidney disease, and cancer.

Take a walk outside. Walking in nature — even looking at pictures of nature — gives a quick, temporary boost to your thinking and memory.

Nature engages your attention not as your main focus but as background. That's why you can talk to someone while walking in the park. Being in nature gives your brain a chance to rest and recover. Strolling down a busy street does not have the same effect. Walking is generally good for your brain.

- Aerobic exercises like fast walking increases brain size in older adults.

- Activity at any age cuts your risk of Alzheimer's disease, even if you're already over 80 years old.

- Exercise could protect you from long-term memory loss after an illness or injury.

Get out there and go for a stroll in the woods or the park, or simply sit outside surrounded by flowers and trees. You'll give your mind a much-needed rest.

Get better sleep. Getting too little sleep on a regular basis ages your brain faster and may raise your risk of Alzheimer's.

Sleep benefits your regular memory, too. The next time you're trying to learn something, practice it right before bedtime. Sleeping right after you learn something helps you retain it better.

Getting a full night's sleep after learning improved people's episodic memory (the ability to remember events) and their semantic memory (the ability to remember facts).

"Since we found that sleeping soon after learning benefited both types of memory, this means that it would be a good thing to rehearse any information you need to remember just prior to going to bed," suggests Notre Dame psychologist and study author Jessica Payne. "In some sense, you may be 'telling' the sleeping brain what to consolidate."

Free games that stretch your brain

So you don't have a buddy nearby to play chess or Scrabble? Nowadays, you don't need one. If you have a computer, you can find game programs like Solitaire and Chess where you can play solo against the machine.

Prefer playing with real people? Make new friends online with games like "Words with Friends" and "Chess with Friends," both offered for free at *www.zyngawithfriends.com*. Enlist your old friends or make new ones, and play from your iPhone or Android smartphone.

Quick tricks to get rid of headaches

Don't let a headache banish you to bed all day. These clever tips can help tame both tension headaches and migraines.

Cross your arms. Crossing your hands over your midsection interferes with your brain's ability to tell where pain is coming from. It may not banish pain permanently, but it may dull or relieve it temporarily.

Massage your skull. People whose migraines are linked to their occipital nerve may score relief with self-massage. Gently work your fingers at the base of your skull. This may relieve migraine pain for a short time, especially if that area tends to feel tender during the headache.

Sip some caffeine. Drinking an 8-ounce cup of coffee after taking ibuprofen can help deliver headache relief. A review of 19 studies found that drinking roughly one cup of coffee alongside a dose of ibuprofen or acetaminophen helped more people find pain relief. Caffeine may give the pain medicine a little extra oomph.

Brew a cup of tea. Specifically, green tea. Then add a fresh sprig of peppermint or spearmint to your cup to tame a tension headache. Or brew a green tea bag and a mint tea bag together for a fast pain fighter.

Try a supplement. People who took a liquid supplement of feverfew and ginger, called LipiGesic, at the first sign of mild headache were less likely to develop a full-blown migraine two hours later. Migraine sufferers squeezed a dose of the liquid under their tongue, held it there for one minute, then took a second dose five minutes later. Those who still had a headache an hour later took two more doses. At the end of two hours, two-thirds of the migraine sufferers were either completely pain-free or had only a mild headache.

You can buy LipiGesic over the counter at your local Walgreens or CVS pharmacy. You can also print coupons from the website *www.lipigesic.com.* Or brew your own homemade ginger and feverfew tea.

Avoid it altogether. Prevention is always the best cure. A team of experts in Italy may have found a way to halt daily tension headaches with a few stretches. They tested their techniques on more than 900 people. After six months of simple, daily stretches and posture exercises, people had fewer headaches and less neck and shoulder pain. Now you can practice these same tricks yourself.

- Sit in an armchair in a quiet room. Apply a heating pad to your shoulders and cheeks. Let your jaw drop naturally in a relaxed position. Do this for 10 to 15 minutes once or twice a day.

- Stand with your back, head, and hands against a wall. Pull your shoulders back until they touch the wall, then release them. Do this eight to 10 times in a row every two or three hours.

- Stand in the same position against the wall. Move your head forward, keeping the rest of your body still, then pull it back again until it touches the wall. Do this eight to 10 times every two to three hours.

- Place your hands behind your neck and lace your fingers together. Tip your head back while gently pulling forward on your neck until you feel a nice stretch. Hold this position for two or three seconds, then relax. Repeat this eight to 10 times, every two or three hours.

The more people stuck to the exercise schedule, the greater relief they felt. Help yourself remember to do the exercises by placing sticky notes around your house. For starters, stick one on your coffee pot, television, and bathroom mirror.

Little-known signs of a migraine

You can spot infamous migraine symptoms like nausea, vomiting, and noise and light sensitivity. But what about yawning or food cravings? Pay attention to these lesser-known signals. You may be able to head off your headache before it starts.

- trouble speaking
- excessive yawning
- blurred vision
- dizziness
- difficulty concentrating
- fatigue
- pale face
- problems reading and writing
- feeling more emotional than usual
- confusion, trouble thinking clearly
- frequent urination
- excessive thirst
- irritability and crankiness
- stiff neck
- food cravings, especially for foods that seem to "trigger" your migraines

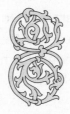

Simple steps to better living

9 phone calls that could save your life

Improving your health can be as easy as picking up the telephone. For emergencies, of course, you can dial "911." But the following calls get a "ringing" endorsement anytime.

Dial your dentist. Make an appointment to get your teeth cleaned, and you'll have plenty of reasons to smile. Your teeth will sparkle, your breath will feel fresh — and you may reduce your risk of heart attack and stroke.

That's what a recent Taiwanese study found. Researchers tracked more than 100,000 people for an average of seven years. Those who regularly got their teeth professionally scraped and cleaned had a 24 percent lower risk of heart attack and a 13 percent lower risk of stroke compared to those who did not.

The link could be inflammation, which plays a role in both gum disease and heart disease. Cleaning your teeth helps eliminate inflammation-causing bacteria.

Make time for a mammogram. Call to schedule a mammogram, and help yourself beat breast cancer. A recent Dutch study found that regular mammograms may reduce the risk of breast cancer deaths by 49 percent. Women ages 70-75 saw a whopping 84 percent lower risk with regular screening.

Mammograms help catch breast cancer early, when the odds of survival are better. By the time cancer was detected in those who didn't get screened, it tended to be more advanced — and deadlier.

Phone a friend. Take a break from making medical appointments, and call a close chum or family member. A friendly chat can be fantastic for your overall well-being.

Studies suggest that social connections help your health in a variety of ways. They may help ward off depression, boost your immune system, lower your blood pressure, and reduce chronic stress, which has been linked to several health problems, including type 2 diabetes and brain shrinkage. On the other hand, loneliness has the opposite effect, increasing depression, anxiety, anger, heart disease, and sleep disturbances.

One University of Michigan study found that a friendly 10-minute talk can boost your brain function, including short-term memory and focus. Stay sharp as you age by staying connected with friends and family.

Take time to help others. You can also connect with strangers in need. Call a worthy organization and offer your services as a volunteer. When you help other people, you also help yourself.

Older folks who volunteer tend to live longer and consider themselves healthier. Volunteering has also been linked to improved mental function, reduced stress, and less depression. It's also a great way to meet new friends who share a common purpose.

Chances are your community has plenty of worthwhile charities that could use your help. To find volunteer opportunities near you, visit VolunteerMatch at *www.volunteermatch.org*, or contact Senior Corps at *www.seniorcorps.gov* or 800-942-2677.

Get technical support from your grandkids. Need help getting online? Call one of your grandkids or a tech-savvy buddy for help. Once you're connected to the Internet, you'll have access to a whole world of information and entertainment. Thanks to new technology, you can:

- find free brainteasers and stimulating online games to keep your mind sharp.

- discover new, high-tech ways to connect to others, including text messaging, email, Facebook, Twitter, and Skype.

- try virtual reality-enhanced exercise, which researchers determined had even more cognitive benefits than regular exercise. People in the study performed "cyber-cyling," which involves pedaling an exercise bike with an interactive screen.

Join a health club. You could also exercise the old-fashioned way — and a gym membership can help keep you motivated. Regular exercise not only keeps you fit, it also plays a key role in fighting heart disease, high blood pressure, high cholesterol, diabetes, dementia, depression, obesity, and other health conditions.

Call a local gym or health club and ask about its rates, hours, and equipment. It may even offer a discount for seniors.

If you are 65 or older, look into the SilverSneakers Fitness Program. Benefits include a free membership at a participating fitness center and exercise classes geared to seniors. Leading Medicare health plans and Medicare Supplement carriers offer the program at no extra cost. For more information, call 888-423-4632 or visit *www.silversneakers.com*.

Call a chimney sweep. A fireplace can keep you warm and toasty, but watch out for chimney fires. They can cost you your home — or even your life. Often, the culprit is soot and creosote buildup inside the chimney.

Arrange for a professional chimney sweep to come for an inspection and cleaning. Just don't expect him to sing "Chim Chim Cher-ee" like Dick Van Dyke in *Mary Poppins*.

Request a radon test. While you're making your home safer, contact a contractor to come test for radon. This colorless, odorless, tasteless gas can seep into your home — especially your basement — from the soil. Prolonged exposure to radon can lead to lung cancer. In fact, radon ranks as the second leading cause of lung cancer in the United States behind cigarettes.

You can also buy radon testing kits at hardware or home improvement stores. If your home has high levels of radon, consider a radon removal system. Other steps include sealing cracks in the foundation and implementing various venting techniques.

For more information about radon and how to deal with it, go to *www.epa.gov/radon* or call the Radon Hotline at 800-767-7236.

Ask about an alert. Emergencies require a quick response. With a personal emergency response system, you can call for help with a push of a button. These buttons, usually worn on a pendant or wristband, come in handy if you live alone and are at risk for heart attack, stroke, falls, or other health emergencies. But first, you have to call to get one.

Shop around and ask questions. Prices and services vary, and there may be installation fees or monthly charges. Ask about contract commitment, battery range, response time, repair policies, cancellation fees, and staff training. Check with your insurance company to see if the cost may be covered or partially covered.

Examples of these alert systems include Medical Guardian at *www.medicalguardian.com* or 800-668-9200 and Medical Alert at *www.medicalalert.com* or 800-800-2537.

Super ways to start your day

Breakfast may be the most important meal of the day, but it's not the only important part of your morning. Get your day off to a spectacular start with these quick, easy-to-follow tips. They only take a few minutes or so, but their impact will last all day — and beyond. Make these key steps part of your morning routine.

Wake up with a workout. Hit the ground running with some exercise. You may think you don't have the time or the stamina to fit a full workout into your day, but a short workout yields big benefits. The trick is to push yourself hard for just a minute at a time.

Researchers at McMaster University in Canada have studied the impact of brief, high-intensity workouts. In one two-week study of eight older people with type 2 diabetes, this type of workout rapidly lowered blood sugar levels.

Get the 'buzz' on hidden caffeine

Taking a multivitamin or dietary supplement may be part of your morning routine — but you might be getting more than you bargained for. While these pills help provide the nutritional boost you need, they can also give you an unexpected jolt of caffeine.

A study by the U.S. Department of Agriculture examined 53 supplements and found roughly half of them contained as much caffeine as one or two cups of coffee. Some packed a whopping eight cups worth of caffeine.

You may not realize that by looking at the label since it only has to list pure caffeine. But caffeine occurs naturally in several botanicals — such as guarana, yerba mate, kola nut, or green tea extract — that may also be ingredients in your supplements.

Sports nutrition and weight loss supplements are the main culprits, but caffeine can also lurk in some multivitamins and mineral products.

People in the study had three supervised training sessions each week. For each workout, they furiously pedaled a stationary bicycle for a minute, then recovered for a minute. They repeated this pattern for a total of 10 sets. Including a three-minute warmup period and a two-minute cool-down period, each workout lasted a total of 25 minutes. But it featured only 10 minutes of vigorous exercise.

Similar studies by the same researchers have shown benefits for unfit but otherwise healthy people and even people with heart conditions.

You can also opt for a longer, less intense workout if you have the time. But don't wait until after you eat breakfast. The timing of your morning workout could make the difference.

One Belgian study found that people who exercised before breakfast did not gain weight, even though they ate a high-calorie, high-fat diet. Meanwhile, people on the same diet who exercised after breakfast did gain weight.

Exercising in the morning before eating seems to burn more fat, improve glucose tolerance, and spark changes in muscle cells that can lead to improved insulin sensitivity.

However, the study included only physically fit young men, and workouts lasted 60 to 90 minutes and included a combination of running and cycling. Check with your doctor before starting any exercise routine.

Scrub away your stress. After your workout, hop in the shower. As you scrub your body, you'll also wash away your worries. That's what a recent University of Michigan study discovered. Showering — or just washing your hands — helps clean your mind as well. You may doubt your own decisions less and look on the brighter side of bad situations. It's a perfect way to boost your mood and start each day with a clean slate.

Spray your shower. Make sure you also start each day with a clean shower. After your morning shower, spray your shower walls and curtain with a daily shower cleaner. But don't shell out big bucks for commercial cleaning products.

Clean up your shower without cleaning out your wallet. Mix these two common household items to create your own shower spray for pennies. Pour 8 ounces of rubbing alcohol into a 32-ounce spray bottle, and top it off with water. Spray this concoction on all shower surfaces to cut down on soap scum. You don't even have to rinse it off. Keep germs away with this one simple, cheap solution. It will keep mildew off your shower, too.

Take care of your toothbrush. You know you should brush and floss your teeth each day. Clean, white teeth give you a beautiful smile, and smiling at other people all day will make you feel good, too. But your toothbrush can harbor lots of bacteria. Take some steps to keep your toothbrush in tiptop shape.

- Rinse your toothbrush thoroughly after brushing your teeth.

- Let it dry. Do not use a toothbrush cover, which provides a damp, enclosed environment for bacteria to grow.

- Stand it upright in a holder, rather than laying it flat. Do not share a holder with anyone else, since your toothbrushes may touch and swap germs.

- Replace your toothbrush every three to four months.

You can also disinfect your toothbrush with a toothbrush sanitizer. Just make sure you use a product approved by the FDA. Other good tips include washing your hands before brushing your teeth and making sure your toothbrush is not too close to the toilet, which sprays bacteria into the air when flushed.

Slather on some sunscreen. Before you leave the house, put on some sunscreen. It's an easy step to forget if you're not spending the day at the beach. But if you're spending any time outdoors, you should not skip it.

Nearly 70 percent of women make this mistake with their skin, leading to premature aging or even cancer. Discover how to preserve your looks, maybe even your life. It's easy. Just make applying sunscreen part of your morning routine.

New labeling guidelines should make it even easier to get the maximum amount of protection. In addition to an SPF number of at least 15, look for the term "broad spectrum" on labels. This means the product will block both ultraviolet A (UVA) and ultraviolet B (UVB) rays. You'll guard against sunburn, wrinkles, and skin cancers.

One recent Australian study determined that regular use of sunscreen lessens the risk of melanoma, a deadly skin cancer. The key is to apply it daily to your face, neck, arms, and hands. But chances are you're not using enough. One rule of thumb is to use a full ounce of sunscreen, or enough to fill a shot glass. For best results, reapply sunscreen every two hours.

You can even find sunscreen in some cosmetic products, like foundation or moisturizer, but probably not enough to fully protect you. As with regular sunscreen, read labels to make sure you know what you're getting.

Soothe your soul. So far, you've taken care of your body, mind, teeth, skin, and even your toothbrush and shower. But don't neglect your spiritual side. Take a few minutes each morning to pray, read scripture or an inspirational book, or visualize positive aspects of your day.

Focusing on positive feelings like hope, love, forgiveness, and gratefulness can help put you at peace and give you the strength to face life's obstacles.

Studies show that prayer may even help you live longer and recover faster from a variety of physical, psychological, and emotional problems — including heart disease, high blood pressure, anxiety, and depression.

If you know someone battling illness, say a prayer for them, too. Evidence suggests this can help — even if they don't know you're praying for them.

Defeat congestion without drugs

Stuffed up? Breathe easier without making a trip to the drug store. Try these natural remedies to relieve congestion.

- Munch on mandarin oranges. A U.S. Department of Agriculture study found that these juicy fruits contain high levels of synephrine, a natural decongestant.

- Hum a happy tune. Humming increases the airflow between your sinuses and your nasal cavities. This extra ventilation helps you breathe and may lower the risk of infection.

- Sip a soothing tea. Cloves naturally help you cough up mucus, so adding them to your tea speeds recovery. Put two cloves and a cinnamon stick in an infuser, and set it in a large mug with a black tea bag. Pour boiling water into the mug, and let it steep for a minute or two.

- Create a quick-acting concoction. Mix one teaspoon of freshly grated horseradish with one-quarter cup of lemon juice, and drink it for rapid mucus release.

Uncommon ways to conquer the common cold

Achoo! Cold and flu season is nothing to sneeze at. To protect yourself, make sure to get your seasonal flu shot and wash your hands frequently. But don't stop there. Learn surprising ways to boost your immune system, avoid germs, and stay healthy all year round.

Clobber colds with kiwi. Discover the succulent fruit with as much fiber as whole-grain cereal, vitamin C equal to two oranges, and the potassium strength of a banana. Thanks to these and other nutrients, it protects against vision loss, cancer, heart attack, stroke, and chronic constipation — all in a neat little package.

Kiwi, or kiwifruit, gets its name for the flightless national bird of New Zealand. But this tiny, tasty fruit can help you soar past cold symptoms.

One New Zealand study found that eating kiwifruit reduced the severity and duration of certain cold and flu symptoms, such as head congestion and sore throat, in older people. It also boosted blood concentrations of vitamin C. In another study, Swedish researchers reported that a high intake of vitamin C from foods lowered the risk of upper respiratory tract infections in women. As an excellent source of vitamin C, kiwifruit would make a fine addition to your diet.

Strengthen your defenses with sweet potatoes. While you're buying some kiwifruit at the supermarket, stay in the produce aisle and grab a sweet potato as well. It's fresh, inexpensive, and boosts immunity while slowing down the aging process.

That's because it provides plenty of beta carotene, an antioxidant that zaps harmful free radicals and which your body converts to vitamin A. High blood levels of beta carotene may reduce your risk of infections like the common cold.

Carotenoids, including beta carotene, may even fight wrinkles, according to a German study. Eating more sweet potatoes is an easy way to get more carotenoids in your diet.

Sweet potatoes are easy to cook, too. Just pop them in the oven to bake. You can also peel them, cut them into wedges, and roast them with some olive oil on a baking sheet. Or make mashed sweet potatoes for a colorful change of pace. For best results, add a little butter or olive oil. A touch of fat helps your body metabolize vitamin A.

Swab suspect surfaces. Public places pose their share of cold and flu risks, but germs also lurk right in your own home. Think of areas touched often, by multiple sets of hands. Regularly wash doorknobs, light switches, and telephones with disinfectant. This simple monthly habit will help to keep colds and flu at bay. It's an easy, but effective, way to minimize your risk — and your trips to the doctor's office.

Other popular germ hideouts in your home include television remote controls, bathroom taps, and refrigerator doors. Make sure to give them a regular wipe as well.

Surprising spots for germs

Your next restaurant meal may come with a heaping side of germs. Menus, fast food trays, and condiment dispensers can all harbor the bugs that cause colds and flu. To protect yourself, make sure your menu doesn't touch your silverware or plate, and wash your hands after ordering.

While you're out and about, beware of these other spots where germs tend to gather.

- pens at banks and shopping malls
- magazines at the doctor's office
- ATM keypads
- gas pump handles
- crosswalk buttons
- vending machine buttons
- grocery cart handles

And don't forget your own pocketbook or cellphone. Be careful where you set these items down. Antibacterial wipes can help remove germs from your phone. But three swipes with a clean, wet tissue can be just as effective.

Beware of germ hotspots. Next time you hunt for bargains at the mall, you might come home with more than a few shopping bags. You could easily catch a cold.

Shopping malls aren't just packed with stores — they're loaded with germs. Food court tables, escalator handrails, toy stores and gadget shops where people handle the merchandise, and makeup samples are some of the biggest culprits.

Of course, so is the restroom. Public restrooms, whether located in a mall or not, feature a smorgasbord of dangers. Germs can lurk on the sink, door handles, and even the soap dispenser.

You know you should wash your hands thoroughly, but make sure to dry them properly, too. If the restroom has a dryer, don't rub your hands together under it. This could dislodge bacteria deep in your pores. Instead, keep your palms under the dryer for at least 30 seconds.

Try out unusual products. While you're at the mall, look for new products that promise to fight off colds and flu. Options include nose products like Nozin Nasal Sanitizer, a mix of alcohol antiseptic and moisturizer you apply around and just inside your nostrils, and GermBullet, a blend of 11 oils in an inhaler. You may also find GermBana antibacterial scarves and other winter gear designed to stop you from spreading germs or catching them from others.

Measure the perfect amount. If you do happen to get sick and need to take medicine, make sure you're doing it right. Do not rely on kitchen spoons to measure liquid medicine. A Cornell study found that using a kitchen spoon led to either pouring an average of 8 percent too little or 12 percent too much medicine, depending on the size of the spoon. Use a proper device, like a measuring cap, dropper, dosing spoon, or syringe to make sure you get the right amount of medicine.

Reap extra benefit from flu vaccine

Getting the seasonal flu vaccine each year may do more than help you ward off the flu. A British study found that the flu shot also cut the risk of heart attack by 19 percent in people ages 40 and older. Early birds reap even more protection, as those who got vaccinated early in flu season — from September to mid-November — lowered their risk by 21 percent. Those who waited until later reduced their risk by only 12 percent.

Sidestep scary side effects of everyday drugs

Modern medicine can help relieve pain, treat chronic conditions, and extend your life. But with so many drugs on the market, some important details get lost in the fine print. Several commonly used prescription and over-the-counter drugs can cause surprising problems. Here's how to protect yourself from these little-known dangers.

Boost your levels of key nutrients. Every battle has its casualties, and the battle for your health is no different. Drugs provide protection, but that protection comes with a price. Over time, some drugs can blunt how your body absorbs, uses, or stores key nutrients.

Make room for must-eat foods if you're taking meds for cholesterol, arthritis, or diabetes. They replenish the nutrients your prescriptions may be sapping, helping you feel better and live longer. Here's a quick look at the culprits.

- Cholesterol-lowering drugs. Often prescribed to bring down high cholesterol, statins also reduce levels of coenzyme Q10 (CoQ10) in your body. Because CoQ10 plays an important role in energy production, low levels can leave you feeling weak and fatigued. They can also lead to heart failure.

To boost your CoQ10 levels, you will likely need to take supplements under a doctor's supervision. But you can also find small amounts of CoQ10 in beef, chicken, mackerel, bran, sesame, beans, spinach, sardines, and peanuts.

- Arthritis drugs. Anti-inflammatory drugs may soothe arthritis pain, but they can also steal key nutrients. Nonsteroidal anti-inflammatory drugs (NSAIDs) can deplete levels of folic acid, while corticosteroids may leave you with less than ideal amounts of vitamins A, C, D, B6, B12, and folic acid and lower levels of minerals like calcium, magnesium, chromium, potassium, selenium, and zinc.

  Taking a multivitamin and multimineral supplement can help. So can making sure your diet contains plenty of salads and whole grains to get the vitamins and minerals you need.

- Diabetes drugs. Oral hypoglycemic drugs, which help control blood sugar in people with type 2 diabetes, may deplete levels of vitamin B12, folic acid, and CoQ10. That's troubling because your pancreas needs CoQ10 to help make insulin. Again, make sure you eat foods that replace these key nutrients.

Eat a medication-friendly menu. Just as drugs can affect your nutrients, the foods you eat can affect your drugs. Some foods interfere with drugs, either enhancing or decreasing the drugs' powers. You could end up not getting enough of the medicine you need — or even overdosing on it.

One combination to avoid is statins and certain fruit juices, including grapefruit, pomegranate, and cranberry. They will cause your body to absorb too much of the drug. Dairy products can limit the effect of certain antibiotics. And leafy greens, rich in vitamin K, can counteract the effects of the blood-thinning drug warfarin.

Coffee may reduce the absorption of some drugs, including thyroid medications and osteoporosis drugs. Meanwhile, other drugs, such as antidepressants and antibiotics, may enhance the effects of coffee. These drugs block an enzyme that helps metabolize caffeine, keeping it in your system longer.

Check meds for unwelcome surprise

Vegetarians go to great lengths to avoid eating animal products. But here's some beastly news — you might be taking them in through your medication.

Tablets and liquid medicines often contain gelatin, which is derived from animal bones or skin. While not an active ingredient in the medicine, gelatin helps hold tablets and capsules together or thicken liquids. Generic drugs, especially, tend to use gelatin during the manufacturing process.

This can come as an unwelcome surprise. In a recent British study, about one-quarter of people who said they preferred not to eat animal products were already taking drugs that contained gelatin.

In some cases, there is no alternative. But if you're concerned about avoiding animal products, ask your doctor or pharmacist if your pills contain any. You may be able to swap your current medication for a "meatless" option.

Get familiar with your painkillers. Your head, back, or muscles hurt, and you need something to relieve the pain. But what over-the-counter option should you choose? What's the difference between ibuprofen, acetaminophen, and aspirin? Plenty.

- Ibuprofen is a nonsteroidal anti-inflammatory drug (NSAID), which means it fights pain by reducing inflammation. Examples include Advil and Motrin. Ibuprofen acts quickly and does not stay in your body for long, making it one of the lower-risk NSAIDs.

- Aspirin belongs to the NSAID group, but it also boasts anti-clotting properties. This makes it a good weapon against heart attack and stroke. High doses of aspirin come with a risk of bleeding, so it may not be the best choice for pain relief.

While both ibuprofen and aspirin have their benefits, taking them together may be deadly. A University of Buffalo study found that ibuprofen lessens aspirin's anti-clotting powers, which could lead to a stroke. Lab tests and other studies yield similar results. Taking ibuprofen and other arthritis drugs like naproxen and celecoxib, along with low-dose aspirin, may counteract aspirin's heart-protective effects.

One possible solution is to take aspirin at least half an hour before taking ibuprofen. Let your doctor know you're taking aspirin before being prescribed any pain medication.

- Acetaminophen, unlike ibuprofen and aspirin, is not an NSAID and works to relieve pain in different ways. That makes it gentler on the stomach than NSAIDs. The active ingredient in Tylenol, acetaminophen also reduces fever.

Unfortunately, it may also blunt the effectiveness of your flu shot. A Czech study found that giving infants acetaminophen weakened the immune response to the flu vaccine. While those who got acetaminophen had fewer fevers — a common reaction to immunization — they also produced fewer anti-bodies to fight off infection.

Animal studies suggest that other pain relievers, including NSAIDs like aspirin, ibuprofen, and naproxen, have a similar effect. It may be best not to take any of these drugs in the weeks before and after your flu vaccine.

Just because you can get a drug without a prescription doesn't mean it comes without side effects. Your over-the-counter painkiller could damage your kidneys, liver, and brain.

For example, taking a second dose of Tylenol for an extra pain-relief boost could lead to big trouble. A British study found that repeated doses of slightly too much acetaminophen, or "staggered overdoses," can be fatal. Besides liver failure — the main risk of too much acetaminophen — staggered overdoses often resulted in brain damage, kidney failure, and even death.

The most common reason for the staggered overdoses was pain relief. But it's shockingly easy to get too much of this drug even by accident. That's because acetaminophen is an ingredient in several prescription and over-the-counter medications for headaches, colds, flu, allergies, sinus problems, sleeplessness, and pain relief.

To protect your liver and other organs, read labels and dosing instructions carefully. And don't take more than one product containing acetaminophen at a time.

Limit memory-stealing drugs. Remember to ask your doctor about anticholinergic drugs. These kinds of drugs may affect your learning and reasoning abilities and increase your risk of memory loss. That's because they either directly or indirectly block the neurotransmitter acetylcholine, which affects memory and thinking.

The effects of these drugs increase over time, so the more you take, the worse off you'll be. The problem is that many drugs have anticholinergic effects. Those with the strongest effects include Paxil, Benadryl, and oxybutynin, a drug taken for overactive bladder. Others with milder effects include the heart drug digoxin, warfarin, codeine, and prednisone. Even over-the-counter drugs like antihistamines and allergy medications have anticholinergic effects.

Beware of blood pressure changes. Mixing blood pressure medication with antibiotics could land you in the hospital. A Canadian study of people ages 66 or older found that taking calcium-channel blockers, a type of blood pressure-lowering drug, at the same time as certain antibiotics may result in a severe drop in blood pressure or shock that requires hospitalization. The problematic antibiotics were erythromycin and clarithromycin. Another similar antibiotic, azithromycin, did not increase the risk of hypotension, or low blood pressure.

On the other hand, many common prescription and over-the-counter drugs may be underlying causes of high blood pressure, according to a recent Israeli study. These drugs include NSAIDs, antidepressants, corticosteroids, bacterial antibiotics, and anti-vascular endothelial growth factor drugs.

If your medication is causing high blood pressure, your doctor may take you off the drug, lower the dosage, or add a blood pressure-lowering drug to your treatment. In some cases, the benefits of the drug outweigh the risk of elevated blood pressure.

Surprising meds that can send you to the hospital

Painkillers get plenty of attention, but they're not the medications sending seniors to the emergency room. A recent study reported that the blood-thinning drug warfarin accounts for a whopping one-third of all emergency hospitalizations for adverse drug effects. And diabetes medications, particularly insulin, cause big problems for older adults as well.

The study found that more than 99,000 hospitalizations of people over age 65 resulted from dangerous problems with prescription drugs. Two-thirds of all hospitalizations were for unintentional overdoses, others involved allergic reactions, and nearly half involved people age 80 or older. Surprisingly, only 1.2 percent came from medications designated as high-risk, including painkillers.

To minimize your risk, always carefully read the instructions that come with your medication. If you're unclear about anything, ask your doctor or pharmacist.

8 nifty ways to knock out pneumonia

Huey "Piano" Smith's rollicking song "Rockin' Pneumonia And the Boogie Woogie Flu" makes pneumonia sound like a grand old time. But the "rockin' pneumonia" is the only kind of pneumonia you ever want to have. Actual pneumonia is no party. In fact, it leads to over a million hospitalizations and tens of thousands of deaths each year. Older people are especially at risk. Take these simple steps to protect yourself from this potentially deadly condition.

Vanquish it with vaccines. Your best shot at preventing pneumonia involves getting shots. Pneumonia is an inflammation of the lungs caused by infection from bacteria, viruses, or other organisms. Getting vaccinated helps guard against these infections.

Experts recommend that everyone age 65 or older get the following two vaccines:

- pneumococcal vaccine, which protects against *Strepto-coccus pneumoniae*, a common bacterial cause of pneumonia. While this vaccine was previously a one-time shot, current recommendations suggest you get a booster shot every five years if you were first vaccinated before you turned 65.

- seasonal flu shot, which helps stave off the influenza viruses that cause flu. If you get the flu, your immune system becomes weakened — and ripe for pneumonia. Get a flu shot each fall. They're available at your doctor's office, walk-in clinics, drugstores, and even some grocery stores.

Prevent it with cereal. Start your day with a bowl of whole-grain cereal, the one food that protects you from heart attack, pneumonia, and infections. People who eat it live longer, too. And you can get it at the corner grocery.

A recent study found that a high intake of dietary fiber — especially the kind found in whole grains — reduced the risk of death from a variety of causes, including heart disease, respiratory diseases like pneumonia, and infectious diseases.

Fiber may work by slashing blood fats, keeping blood sugar steady, lowering blood pressure, and fighting inflammation. The anti-inflammatory powers may account for its positive effect on respiratory illnesses, like pneumonia.

Look for a high-fiber cereal made with whole grains. It could be the most important meal you eat all day. Other good sources of whole-grain fiber include oatmeal, popcorn, wheat germ, brown rice, bran, and whole-grain breads.

Zap it with zinc. This important mineral may help keep pneumonia at bay. That's because it plays a key role in maintaining your immune system.

One study of older people living in nursing homes in the Boston area found that those with low zinc levels have a higher risk of pneumonia. Compared to those with low levels, people with normal zinc levels had fewer cases of pneumonia, and their bouts of pneumonia were shorter. They also needed about half as many antibiotic prescriptions and boasted a lower death rate.

Researchers suspect that poor zinc status impairs your immune response, which makes you more susceptible to infections like pneumonia.

Ask your doctor about zinc supplements. You can also find zinc in plenty of foods, including oysters, red meat, shellfish, lima beans, peanut butter, and several breakfast cereals. Zinc lozenges and nasal gels may also help fight off colds.

Defeat it with vitamin D. Keep your lungs in tiptop shape, so they can better withstand an infection. Boosting your vitamin D levels may help your lungs work better.

New Zealand researchers have linked higher blood levels of vitamin D to better lung function. Specifically, the study measured forced expiratory volume, or FEV, and forced vital capacity, or FVC. FEV measures how much air you can breathe out in one second while FVC measures how much you can blow out after taking a deep breath then exhaling as quickly as possible. People with higher blood levels of vitamin D had better results on both breathing tests.

While the study does not prove a clear cause-and-effect relationship, it can't hurt to boost your vitamin D levels.

Your body naturally produces vitamin D from sunlight, but this ability declines with age. Still, spending some more time in the sun can help.

You can also get vitamin D from supplements and fortified foods, including milk, orange juice, and breakfast cereals. Natural food sources of vitamin D include liver, egg yolks, and oily fish like salmon, mackerel, tuna, and sardines.

Tackle it with tea. Sip green tea, and you just might strengthen your defenses against pneumonia. Japanese researchers found that women who drank five or more cups of green tea a day were 47 percent less likely to die of pneumonia. Just drinking about a cup of tea each day lowered the risk by 41 percent. That's because the antioxidants in tea may fight off viruses and other harmful microorganisms.

To make the most of green tea, drink regular tea rather than the decaffeinated kind. Decaf tea has fewer catechins, the antioxidant flavonoids that give green tea its healing powers. Instead of milk or cream, add lemon juice or another type of citrus juice to your tea. The acidic nature of the citrus juice will help more catechins survive the trip through your digestive system so you can reap their benefits.

Ward if off by washing your hands. It may not be the most exciting mode of defense, but it's among the most effective. Regularly washing your hands helps defend against germs that can lead to flu or pneumonia. Don't feel like you need to spring for fancy antibacterial solutions, either. Plain old soap and water will do.

Try not to cough or sneeze into your hands. Opt for a tissue or the crook of your elbow instead. To further fight germs, use antibacterial wipes on phones, computer keyboards, the television remote control, and other surfaces you often touch.

Germs can pop up in unexpected places — like the 3-D glasses in movie theaters. To protect yourself, clean the glasses with a disinfectant wipe or with soap and water from the restroom. Don't rely on wiping them with a dry tissue. That will only get rid of about two-thirds of the germs.

Beat it by brushing and flossing. Good hygiene shouldn't stop with your hands. Take care of your teeth and gums, too. Gum problems have been linked to pneumonia and other respiratory infections.

In one study, brushing teeth three times a day reduced the risk of pneumonia by up to 50 percent for people on ventilation in the hospital. Ventilation-associated pneumonia is a common problem, because bacteria from the mouth can travel to the lungs and take advantage of the patient's weakened immune system.

Even if you're not hooked up to a ventilator, you should guard your gums. Brush and floss daily, don't avoid the dentist, and treat any gum infections promptly.

Minimize it by monitoring your meds. Some solutions can also be problems. Beware of certain medications that might help treat one condition but put you at higher risk of pneumonia.

Inhaled corticosteroids, often prescribed for chronic obstructive pulmonary disease (COPD), may boost your risk of pneumonia. People taking the highest dose of these drugs and those who have the weakest lungs are most vulnerable.

Acid-suppressing medications, like proton pump inhibitors (PPIs) and histamine 2 receptor antagonists, may also raise your pneumonia risk. That could be because they increase your stomach's pH, making the environment less acidic and allowing bacteria to colonize.

Ask your doctor about alternatives to these medications. Keep in mind that the benefits of the drugs may outweigh the risks. Just use these drugs with caution — and take other steps to reduce your risk of pneumonia.

Swallowing woes boost risk

If you have trouble swallowing, you could be in big trouble. This problem, known as dysphagia, could result in pneumonia.

That's because food particles that end up in your trachea, or windpipe, can make their way to your lungs and foster the growth of bacteria. This could lead to a type of pneumonia called "aspiration pneumonia."

Dysphagia is more common in older people, whose muscles — including those involved in swallowing — have weakened. It could hamper your ability to swallow liquids, food, pills, or even saliva. Warning signs include coughing or gagging while eating or drinking and the feeling that food is getting stuck in your throat.

You can take steps to reduce your risk, such as improving your posture while eating, taking smaller bites, eating more slowly, and chewing thoroughly. Exercises can also help strengthen your tongue, jaw, and lips. See your doctor if you suffer from swallowing problems.

Humble veggie that can change your life

Popeye's secret weapon packs plenty of nutritional punch — and quite a wallop against disease. Find out how spinach can change your life for the better and how you can make the most of this humble vegetable.

Spinach is so packed with key nutrients — including magnesium, vitamin K, vitamin C, vitamin E, folate, fiber, carotenoids, manganese, and antioxidant flavonoids — that just two servings a week is enough to measurably reduce the risk of life-threatening diseases.

For example, Canadian researchers found that men who ate two or more servings of spinach a week reduced their risk of aggressive prostate cancer by 37 percent compared to those who ate spinach less than once a month.

Learn more about spinach's amazing health benefits and discover helpful tips you can use to boost its power.

Maximize your magnesium. Muscle weakness or spasms, a change in heart rate, headaches, high blood pressure, and more — all can be caused by deficiency of this important mineral. Luckily, spinach helps provide your body with this key nutrient. One-half cup of cooked frozen spinach gives you 78 milligrams (mg) of magnesium. And a little magnesium can go a long way.

- Dodge diabetes. Six months to better blood sugar control — even if you're overweight. All you need is a daily dose of magnesium. That's what German researchers recently discovered.

  In the study, overweight people who received magnesium supplements for six months showed improved blood sugar levels and insulin sensitivity. These results suggest that boosting your magnesium intake may help ward off diabetes. Even if you already have diabetes, magnesium supplements may help.

- Unleash a super antioxidant. You need magnesium to synthesize glutathione, the "sticky" antioxidant that sweeps deadly toxins — including mercury and plastics — from your body. Glutathione works better than vitamins to keep you healthy. Like other antioxidants, glutathione neutralizes harmful free radicals. But this amazing molecule also helps other antioxidants, including vitamin C, work even better. Fresh fruits and veggies, like spinach, help boost glutathione.

- Sidestep stroke. Eating more spinach and other magnesium-rich foods may reduce your risk of stroke. In an analysis of seven previous studies, Swedish researchers determined that every 100-mg increase in dietary magnesium cut the risk of stroke by 8 percent. You can get about 100 mg of magnesium from three-quarters of a cup of cooked spinach. Magnesium may help control your risk of stroke by lowering blood pressure or by reducing the risk of type 2 diabetes, another risk factor for stroke.

KO disease with vitamin K. This underrated anti-aging vitamin may be the key to preventing fragile bones, hardened arteries, heart disease, and cancer. Eat more vitamin K-rich spinach now to feel younger longer.

You need vitamin K for blood clotting, but this vitamin has several other health benefits. A long-term lack of vitamin K may boost your risk of degenerative diseases such as osteoporosis, or brittle bone disease, and atherosclerosis, or hardening of the arteries.

Besides strengthening your bones and protecting your arteries, vitamin K may also reduce the inflammation associated with chronic diseases, such as heart disease and arthritis, and improve insulin sensitivity to help ward off diabetes. One Mayo Clinic study found that dietary vitamin K reduces the risk of non-Hodgkin lymphoma, a cancer of the immune system.

While current FDA guidelines recommend 90 micrograms (mcg) of vitamin K a day for women and 120 mcg a day for men, evidence suggests you should get more. One cup of raw spinach gives you 145 mcg of vitamin K. In addition to spinach, other leafy greens like kale, Swiss chard, collard greens, turnip greens, and mustard greens provide vitamin K.

Easy ways to slip spinach into your diet

Spinach is cheap, nutritious, and beneficial to your health. And, with only seven calories in each cup of raw spinach, it won't balloon your waistline. But don't forget that spinach also tastes great. Here are some easy ways to add more spinach to your meals.

- Make salads with raw spinach. Toss with some nuts, dried fruit, cheese, and vinaigrette for added flavor and texture.

- Put spinach leaves instead of lettuce on your sandwiches.

- Sauté, boil, or braise spinach to make a scrumptious side dish.

- Cooking spinach really concentrates the nutrients — but remember to cook more than you think you'll need, since a pound will dwindle down to about a cup after cooking.

- Spice things up. Don't like the taste of cooked spinach? Add garlic, parmesan cheese, balsamic vinegar, or nutmeg to jazz it up.

- Rethink your recipes. Add spinach to pasta dishes, casseroles, dips, soups, and egg dishes.

Pick the right package. One cup of raw spinach only costs about 52 cents, which is quite a bargain. Shed some light on your spinach, and you'll get even more bang for your buck.

Fluorescent light, like the kind used in supermarkets, may boost the nutrients in spinach, making it more nutritionally dense than spinach stored in the dark. That's because artificial lighting mimics sunlight and triggers photosynthesis, leading to more vitamin C, vitamin E, vitamin K, and folate.

Choose packages of spinach near the front of the produce bin, where there's more light. But make sure to examine the spinach carefully. More exposure to light could also lead to more wilting.

Store it with smarts. Once you buy your spinach, make sure it doesn't spoil before you get a chance to eat it. As produce ripens, it emits ethylene, a gas that speeds up spoilage. Store raw spinach in its original packaging in the crisper drawer of your refrigerator. Although the bag may look solid, it should let ethylene escape.

For spinach that doesn't come with packaging, put the unwashed leaves in an open plastic bag in the crisper. You can wrap a paper towel around the spinach to help absorb moisture. Use spinach within a week.

Heed these red flags — or else

You don't want to run to the doctor's office for every sniffle, cough, or minor ache or pain. But some symptoms require swift action. That's because they could be early signs of a dangerous illness. Although your instinct may be to wait or tough it out, that approach could put your health — and even your life — at risk. Pay attention to the following warning signs. And ignore them at your own peril.

Stand up to dizziness. Feel dizzy or lightheaded when you stand up? It could be because of a drastic drop in blood pressure. Called "orthostatic hypotension," this plunge happens when you move from a reclining to an upright position. It can make you feel dizzy or even faint. Even worse, it could mean a higher risk of heart failure.

That's what a recent study discovered. Researchers measured participants' blood pressure when they were lying down and after they stood. If their systolic blood pressure, or top number, dropped by 20 or more points or if the diastolic blood pressure, or bottom number, dropped by 10 or more points, then they were considered to have this condition.

Over more than 17 years of follow-up, those with orthostatic hypotension were 54 percent more likely to develop heart failure. Even after excluding people with high blood pressure — because that also heightens your risk — people with this type of dizziness had a 34-percent greater risk of heart failure. The link was especially strong for people ages 45 to 55.

Not every dizzy spell means your heart is in jeopardy, but if you often feel dizzy upon standing, you should mention this to your doctor.

Take note of tremors. Most people realize that persistent tremors could be a sign of Parkinson's disease. But most people employ some pretty shaky logic when it comes to reporting these symptoms to their doctor.

In a survey by the National Parkinson Foundation, 61 percent of men and 55 percent of women said they would wait rather than see their doctor right away. That's a mistake, because getting early treatment can make a difference.

Other early warning signs of Parkinson's disease include shaking, trouble walking or walking in a stooped manner, loss of facial expression, dizziness, fainting, trouble sleeping, loss of smell, small handwriting, constipation, and speaking in an unusually soft or low voice.

Report shortness of breath. Huffing and puffing is fine if you're the Big Bad Wolf. Otherwise, it should be cause for alarm. You

When pain should be taken seriously

Aches and pains crop up now and then. But not all pain is created equal.

Seek help for severe headache. Sudden, severe head pain could mean more than a migraine. It could signal a brain aneurysm, a ruptured blood vessel in your brain.

Aspirin won't do any good for this unbearable pain. You need to call 911 or get to an emergency room right away. Once there, a CT scan will determine if there's hemorrhaging, or bleeding in the brain. It might require surgery to stop the bleeding and repair the blood vessel. Quick action is essential, since brain damage can occur within minutes.

Sidestep side discomfort. Do not shrug off that sharp pain in your right side. It could be appendicitis, or inflammation of the appendix.

If the piercing pain in your side worsens and you feel nauseous and feverish, get it checked out right away. You may need to have emergency surgery to remove the inflamed appendix. Leave it alone, and it may burst.

Beware of back numbness. Taking a low-key approach to lower back pain may not be the best move. See a doctor if your aching back also feels numb or the pain travels down the back of your legs — down to your tingling toes. This type of numbing pain could indicate a herniated, or slipped, disc pressing on your spinal nerve.

Most likely, you can treat the problem with a combination of rest, painkillers, and physical therapy. But if these remedies don't work, you may need surgery.

might think you're just old and out of shape, so frequent shortness of breath is only natural — but you'd be wrong.

Shortness of breath can be a sign of serious heart or lung problems — including heart attack, heart failure, asthma, chronic obstructive pulmonary disease (COPD), bronchitis, pneumonia, or even lung cancer. It could also be hyper-ventilation triggered by anxiety.

When it comes to shortness of breath, don't wait a long time to see a doctor — especially if it happens regularly, gets worse, or strikes when you're performing activities that used to pose no problems.

Also let your doctor know if you've had to give up any activities because they used to cause shortness of breath. Often, people neglect to mention this during a doctor's appointment since they no longer experience any symptoms. But this only makes it harder to detect the underlying problem.

Look after your leg. When your leg feels painful and swollen, don't just sit there. That's probably what caused the trouble in the first place. Go to the doctor instead. You may have deep vein thrombosis (DVT), or a blood clot that forms in the veins of your legs.

This condition often occurs when you sit for hours at a time — like during long airplane flights or long hours working at your desk. Besides pain and swelling, other telltale signs of DVT include redness and warmth.

Massaging your sore leg may seem like a good idea, but it's not. In fact, rubbing the area could cause the clot to break free and travel through your bloodstream, where it could do all sorts of damage. If your doctor determines you have DVT, you will probably need to take blood thinners to dissolve the clot.

Bring up bloating. Your belly has certainly felt better. Feeling bloated and gassy now and then should not be cause for alarm. But if you experience bloating, abdominal pain, and trouble eating almost every day for a few weeks, it could be an early sign of ovarian cancer.

You may be at higher risk for ovarian cancer if you have a family history of breast or ovarian cancer or if you've never been pregnant.

Make an appointment with your gynecologist to discuss your persistent bloating and discomfort. Scans can help determine if you have a tumor. The key is to catch this cancer early because survival rates are much better for women who receive an early diagnosis.

Treat tender teeth. Bite into something cold, like ice cream, and you may get a chilly reception from your teeth. If you feel a throbbing or twinge of pain, it could mean that one of your teeth has a damaged nerve. A crack in your tooth may be the culprit. Even worse, this exposed nerve can open the door to bacterial infection — which can affect not only your mouth but also spread throughout your body.

Go to a dentist and have it checked out. You may simply need to get a cavity filled to protect the nerve. But, in the case of infection, you may need a root canal or antibiotics.

Quench your thirst. Refilling your water glass over and over? Hot weather, physical exertion, and other factors can boost your thirst. But increased thirst can also be an early sign of type 2 diabetes. Thirst for some answers, and let your doctor know. A blood glucose screening can help detect the problem early.

Other diabetes warning signs include frequent urination, fatigue, and blurred vision. Being overweight, older, and inactive boosts your risk. So does having high blood pressure or a family history of the disease.

Keep an eye on your vision. Look out! Telltale changes in vision may signal a detached retina. You may see "floaters," which look like spots or hairs floating across your field of vision, or sudden flashes of light. It may also look as if a shadow or curtain has fallen across part of your field of vision.

Left untreated, retinal detachment can lead to permanent vision loss in the affected eye. Luckily, acting quickly can help save your sight. Go to an eye specialist as soon as you notice these warning signs.

Slam the brakes on hidden car dangers

Fasten your seat belt. Your next drive just might make you sick. Discover some of your car's little-known health risks — and how to protect yourself from them.

Obvious driving dangers include bad weather, mechanical breakdowns, blown tires, accidents, reckless or drunk drivers, or drivers distracted by talking or sending text messages on their cell phones. But those are just the dangers you know about. Others lurk in unexpected places.

For example, simply inhaling that exciting "new car smell" may pose a threat. That's because the exhilarating scent is actually produced by a blend of toxic chemicals that "off-gas," or evaporate, from materials in the vehicle's interior. While there's not much you can do about new car smell, you can take these steps to prevent your current car from making you sick.

Vacuum very well. Pet allergens and dust mites could be hiding on your car seats — even if you don't have pets. Wright State University researchers found that most cars contained high enough levels of dog and cat allergens to trigger allergy symptoms.

When vacuuming your car seats, make sure to clean between the seats as well. That's where crumbs can fall, providing a perfect spot — dark and tiny — for bacteria to grow. Food spills are the number one spot for germs in your car, so clean them up as soon as possible. Or refrain from eating in your car in the first place.

And don't forget your car mats. Who knows what bacteria the bottoms of your shoes pick up from the ground and track into your car. To make it easier to clean these mats, swap your carpet mats for removable rubber ones. That way, you can wash them with soap and water.

Disinfect the dash. Your car's dashboard can be a smorgasbord of bacteria and mold. When vents suck in air, they also allow bacteria and mold spores to enter your car. They make themselves at home on the dashboard and thrive in the warm, sunny environment. In fact, besides food spills, your dashboard is the germiest spot in your car.

Keep antibacterial wipes handy and wipe down the dashboard regularly. While you're at it, give the steering wheel and door handles a good wipe, too.

Store medications safely. Going on a trip? Don't stick your medications in your suitcase in the trunk. You don't want them exposed to extreme heat or cold. Otherwise, they may become less effective or even threaten your health. Most medications — other than those that require refrigeration — remain safe within a temperature range of 59 to 86 degrees Fahrenheit. Ideally, keep them between 68 and 77 degrees.

When traveling, put your meds in your purse or a separate bag in the passenger area of your car. Make sure to take the bag with you when you leave the car parked in the sun. When picking up your drugs from the pharmacy on extremely hot or cold days, go straight home.

Shield yourself from the sun. Think you're safe from the sun while you're in your car? Think again. While laminated windshields keep out the sun's ultraviolet (UV) rays, your side and rear windows do not offer the same protection. They only block UVB rays — the kind that cause sunburn — but let in UVA rays, which may boost your risk of skin cancer.

To be safe, apply sunscreen or wear long sleeves when driving or riding for hours in the sun. You can also get your car windows professionally treated to keep out harmful ultraviolet rays.

Find the right fluid. Water may be good enough for your bath or shower but not for your car's windshield. A preliminary British study found that not adding "screenwash," or washer fluid, to your wiper fluid may put you at risk for Legionnaires' disease.

That's likely because *legionella* bacteria could grow in the stagnant water in the windshield wiper fluid holder. When you spray that water on your windshield, some of it may be sucked through the vents, where you can inhale the harmful bacteria. Always put windshield washer fluid — not plain water — in your car's windshield wiper fluid reservoir.

Take these simple precautions, and you'll make a detour around unexpected roadblocks on the road to a long and healthy life.

Heal yourself with humor

It may sound like a funny way to stay healthy, but laughter is no joke. Research shows that laughing can seriously improve your health. Find out how chuckling, giggling, cackling, and guffawing may help you live longer.

Improve blood flow. Loosen up with laughter, and your blood vessels will do the same. That's what researchers at the University of Maryland School of Medicine discovered.

In one study, when people watched scenes from a funny movie, their blood vessels expanded, improving blood flow. On the other hand, watching stressful scenes from a dramatic film caused blood vessels to constrict, impeding blood flow.

The contrast between the conditions was stark, with a 30- to 50-percent difference in blood vessel diameter. Researchers noted that the improvement is similar to the beneficial effects of aerobic exercise or the use of statins.

A pair of studies at the University of Texas yielded similar results. In both studies, participants watched 30 minutes of either a comedy or a disturbing documentary.

Those who watched the comedy had improved "arterial compliance," the amount of blood that flows through your arteries at a given time. That's important because decreased arterial compliance has been linked to high blood pressure and heart disease.

In the other study, the comedy watchers' blood vessels dilated by 21 percent, while the blood vessels of those who watched the documentary constricted by 18 percent. Constricted blood vessels can contribute to high blood pressure. Most encouraging, the positive effects of laughter lingered even 24 hours later.

Of course, you don't have to watch comedies to laugh. Japanese researchers found that "laughter yoga," which combines breathing exercises with laughter, helped lower blood pressure.

9 ways to tickle your funny bone

Laugh more often, and you'll have plenty of reasons to smile. Get the last laugh with a longer, healthier, and more fun-filled life. Here are some surefire ways to tickle your funny bone:

- watch funny movies or TV shows

- swap jokes with friends

- read the comics or humorous books

- seek out funny websites or silly YouTube clips

- spend time with people who make you laugh

- connect with your inner child. Spending time around children, like your grandchildren, is a good way to experience joy and laughter.

- try to see the humor in everyday situations

- make yourself laugh. Even if you don't feel especially jolly, force yourself to laugh. A fake laugh can work just as well as a real one.

- practice laughter yoga. Find out more about this funny form of exercise at *www.laughteryoga.org*.

Elevate good cholesterol. High cholesterol is no laughing matter — but laughing may help your heart by boosting levels of HDL, or good cholesterol.

In a yearlong study of people with type 2 diabetes, high blood pressure, and high cholesterol, those who watched 30 minutes of funny movies or sitcoms each day in addition to their standard treatment reaped the benefits.

After just two months, their HDL levels improved. After fourth months, they also lowered blood levels of certain inflammatory chemicals associated with heart disease.

Lower blood sugar. If you have diabetes, you need to take care of your heart — but don't forget about your blood sugar. Luckily, laughter comes in handy for that, too.

A Japanese study found that laughing may help you side-step unhealthy spikes in blood sugar that can follow meals. Laughter seems to work by sparking changes in genes that regulate blood glucose, thus improving glucose tolerance.

Ease pain. Sometimes you might laugh till it hurts. But a little silliness can also help soothe your pain. Laughing may work by contracting and relaxing certain muscles or just by providing a pleasant distraction. But a recent British study sheds more light on what makes laughter such good medicine.

Turns out that laughing triggers the release of endorphins, brain chemicals that act as natural painkillers. Researchers discovered that laughing actually boosts your tolerance for pain. It's the physical act of laughing itself that helps, so a hearty belly laugh or guffaw works better than a slight chuckle.

Boost your brainpower. "What is laughter?" could be the correct "Jeopardy" response to the clue "Best medicine for a better brain."

A recent Northwestern University study found that people performed better in a word association game after watching a stand-up comedy routine rather than news clips. MRI scans of those who watched the funny video showed increased activity in an area of the brain responsible for broadening attention. That's probably how they were suddenly able to find less obvious connections between words to solve the puzzles. Older studies have also suggested that humor improves memory.

Enhance your immune system. Laughter may be contagious, but it may also help you fight off sickness. A series of studies at Loma Linda University explored the effects of "mirthful laughter" on the immune system using blood samples. People who watched a humorous video for an hour boosted the activity of disease-fighting T cells and natural killer cells, which stave off tumors and viral infections.

Burn calories. Give your funny bone a workout, and you just might end up slightly slimmer. Like exercise, laughing burns calories — just not as many.

Vanderbilt University researchers found that laughter boosted heart rate and energy expenditure by 10 to 20 percent. That's about the same rate as light clerical work, writing, or playing cards.

But a little laughter each day can add up. Researchers estimate that 15 minutes of genuine laughter each day can burn up to 40 calories. Over a year, that can mean a loss of more than 4 pounds.

Spark your appetite. Now here's the punch line — all that laughter can make you hungry. Loma Linda researchers found that laughter has the same appetite-stimulating effect as moderate physical exercise.

Specifically, laughing changes the levels of hormones that regulate hunger. After watching a funny video, people had lower levels of leptin, which suppresses appetite, and higher levels of ghrelin, which stimulates hunger.

This funny business can come in handy for older people who don't have much of an appetite and have difficulty exercising.

Squelch stress. When you're laughing, your worries disappear in a hurry. Laughter reduces levels of stress hormones like cortisol and epinephrine and helps you relax. That's important because stress can have a harmful effect on your health, contributing to high blood pressure, heart attack, stroke, memory loss, and other serious conditions.

Laughter — not always the best medicine

If you have chronic obstructive pulmonary disease (COPD), laughing may do more harm than good. COPD includes both chronic bronchitis and emphysema. Symptoms include wheezing, a chronic cough that brings up phlegm, and shortness of breath.

A recent study of COPD and laughter reveals a mixed bag. People with COPD who have a good sense of humor have fewer symptoms of depression and anxiety and a better quality of life. But the actual physical act of laughing can lead to decreased lung function. After watching a humorous video, people with COPD had more trapped air in their lungs, a condition known as hyperinflation.

Researchers aren't sure if laughing has just a short-term impact on your lungs or if the effects accumulate. But to be safe, consider seeing a dramatic film instead of a comedy next time you go to the movies.

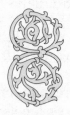

Connect with others to heal body and mind

5 happy habits for brighter days

Stay happy, and you just may live longer. Research shows older people who tend to be in a good mood over the course of a day enjoy a 35 percent lower risk of dying than people who often have bluer moods. The question is — how can you get to that happier place? Here are five habits to cultivate for happier and healthier days.

Start your day with a tasty bowl of cereal. This popular food is naturally low in sodium, saturated fat, and cholesterol. Most enriched cereals like Kellogg's All-Bran and Apple Cinnamon Cheerios can be your diet's top sources of B vitamins, which keep your brain chemicals in balance.

Research that followed 3,503 people 65 years and older for 12 years found that those who got the most vitamin B6 and vitamin B12 had the lowest rates of depression. The U.S. Recommended Daily Allowances for these vitamins are 1.5 milligrams (mg) a day of vitamin B6 and 2.4 micrograms of vitamin B12. You'll get double that amount of both vitamins from a one-half cup serving of All-Bran cereal.

Experts warn that older people tend to be deficient in the B vitamins even more than the rest of the population, so these are nutrients you need to pay attention to. But read the nutrition label on your cereal box to be sure you pick a variety that doesn't have too much fat, sodium, or sugar.

Enjoy a cup of coffee — or make it two. Men who were surveyed said drinking coffee helps motivate them to get a job done, while women said it helps them relax. Whatever your definition of "feeling good," a cup of coffee can help you maintain a good mood.

Researchers looked at results from the Nurses' Health Study, following 50,000 women for 10 years. The women were an average of 63 years old at the start of the study. Those who drank as little as two cups of coffee a day had a lower risk of depression than women who drank very little.

Women who drank at least four cups of coffee daily had the best mood protection, up to 20 percent less risk that those who rarely enjoy a cuppa joe. But only caffeinated coffee did the trick.

You can even time your java for the best mood with the least jitters. The caffeine in coffee can wake you up in the morning and make you more alert. It may even exaggerate the effects of natural hormones like adrenaline. But the effects last for only about two hours. Everyone is different, with some people needing two or three cups to feel alert, while others may feel jittery after a single cup.

And be sure to switch to decaf by late afternoon so you don't drink caffeine too close to bedtime. You'll really be in a bad mood if you can't sleep at night.

Perk up your coffee's taste

Even if you've been brewing coffee for decades, you can refine your skills to make a better-tasting cup. Try all four tricks.

- Take coffee off the burner. Do this within 15 minutes of brewing to protect the flavor of your coffee and avoid a burned taste. Put the coffee in a thermos, then heat it up in the microwave later.

- Clean your machine. Mix a quarter cup baking soda into a cup of water, and put it in your empty coffee maker. Run the machine through a full cycle. Rinse and run another cycle with fresh water.

- Brew with eggshells. Mix a teaspoon of crushed shells from hard-boiled eggs into the coffee grounds before brewing to neutralize the acidity and cut the bitterness.

- Store it right. You don't need to keep ground coffee in the freezer, but you do need to put it in an airtight container.

Remember those raindrops on roses. New York researchers studied people with chronic health problems like asthma and heart disease to see if consciously thinking about the good things in their lives — a beautiful sunrise, an upcoming graduation party — might help them take better care of their health. It worked.

People who used positive affirmations or spent time thinking about something that made them happy every day did better at taking their medicine, going on a daily walk, tracking their blood pressure, and other healthy habits, than those in a control group.

Other longevity experts suggest you try to recall happy things with the idea that they will make you smile. Their research shows that baseball players who had big smiles in photos ended up living up to seven years longer than players with smaller or no smiles in photos. The researchers suspect that smiling helps lower your stress.

Count your blessings. The Apostle Paul advised the Thessalonians, "In everything give thanks; for this is God's will for you in Jesus Christ." Those ancient words of wisdom are still good advice if you're looking to be happier.

Now, it's therapists and counselors who may suggest that you write in a gratitude journal or write letters of gratitude, keeping track of events, things, and people you're thankful for.

So at least once a week, write down five things you're grateful for. Researchers found people who do this have more empathy toward others and don't worry as much about small problems or slights. They also tend to have a happier outlook on life.

You may also set aside time to write a letter of gratitude to someone who has helped you. Experts found doing this once a week helped people feel more content with their lives. You don't even need to mail the letters to get the benefit.

Or consider using an electronic tool to track your gratitude daily. Apps — software applications for your smart phone or computer tablet — like Happy Tapper can help you record and organize things you're grateful for. Look for Happy Tapper at *www.happytapper.com* or purchase it for 99 cents at the iTunes store, *www.apple.com/itunes/*.

Get out and play. Researchers who completed a 10-year study of 50,000 older women found that those who exercised the most were 20 percent less likely to suffer from depression than those who were least active, getting less than 10 minutes a day of exercise. The more exercise the better, it seemed, with women in the happiest group getting at least 90 minutes a day of physical activity.

The study also found that spending too much time watching television seemed to lead to unhappiness. Women who spent three or more hours a day in front of the TV had a 13 per cent higher risk of depression than those who watched the least television.

So don't try to make yourself feel better by vegging out on the couch. Instead, get out and be active doing something you enjoy. Active women in the study reported walking, running, bicycling, playing tennis, swimming, doing aerobics or yoga, and even mowing the lawn. It all helped put a skip in their steps.

Warning — inactivity as deadly as smoking

If you don't get any exercise, you're not alone. Experts say about one-third of adults in the world are inactive, and that figure is even higher in Western nations like the United States.

In a recent worldwide study, researchers looked at what happens to people who don't get any physical activity at all, to say nothing of the recommended 150 minutes per week of moderate activity.

They found that inactivity is even more deadly than smoking, statistically speaking. That's because lack of exercise contributes to deaths from heart disease, diabetes, and cancers like colon cancer and breast cancer. That makes it a serious public health problem, blamed for more than 5 million deaths each year.

Change your habits to save your hearing

Nearly one-third of people 60 years and older have at least moderate hearing loss. Losing your hearing does more than just force you to turn up the volume on your television. It may also be linked to serious health problems, like developing dementia or having trouble walking or keeping your balance.

Maybe worse, when you can't hear what other people are saying, you risk becoming isolated and feeling alone. Perhaps you can fake your way through conversations at first, using social cues or reading lips when your hearing starts to go. But as it gets worse, these tricks may not do the trick. Then you may tend to avoid the embarrassment of difficult conversations.

Keep your social connections and your hearing intact. Don't risk your hearing with these five foolhardy habits.

Taking too many OTC pain relievers. Nearly 100 drugs can cause temporary or permanent hearing loss, but it's not a side effect you usually consider. That may explain why common over-the-counter (OTC) pain relievers are the hidden cause of hearing loss that you may never think about.

Pain relievers including aspirin, acetaminophen, and non-steroidal anti-inflammatory drugs (NSAIDs) like ibuprofen were linked to hearing loss among men who took part in the Health Professionals Follow-up Study. This research looked at the health of nearly 27,000 men, tracking what drugs they took regularly and how their hearing fared over 20 years.

Men who used these painkillers regularly, defined by the researchers as at least twice a week, were more likely to have hearing loss. The longer they used the drugs, the worse the problem was. The effect was strongest among men younger than 50 years old.

Earlier research had shown that some painkillers cut blood flow to the cochlea, the part of your ear that converts sound waves into brain signals.

And painkillers are not the only drugs that could be harming your hearing. Some prescription drugs, including the cancer drug cisplatin, certain loop diuretics, and drugs for erectile dysfunction may also lead to hearing loss.

Musical way to prevent hearing loss

Don't give up playing music just because you think nobody wants to hear you. Researchers found that continuing to play a musical instrument over a lifetime protects your brain's ability to detect and process sound. This can help you keep your hearing as you get older.

Both lifetime musicians and people who never learned to play an instrument were tested in a soundproof room. Experts wanted to see how well they could decipher speech with a noisy background, hear different sound frequencies, pick out gaps in sound, and hear increasingly quieter sounds. Folks who played instruments were better at these hearing tasks, suggesting that their brains retained more sound-processing skills.

But it could also simply be that people with better hearing tend to play — and keep playing — musical instruments.

Overusing cellphones and other tiny electronic gadgets. You can't get away from those little handheld electronic devices that keep you connected to friends and family — and even let you enjoy your favorite music on the go. Whether you prefer to spend time with a cellphone or an MP3 music player next to your ear, too much of a good thing can harm your hearing. In the end, moderation is the key.

First, experts say to limit the amount of time you spend talking on a cellphone. Researchers in Austria questioned people to find out whether cellphone use might be causing tinnitus. This persistent ringing, buzzing, or hissing sound can annoy you to no end while it disrupts your sleep and keeps you from concentrating. Tinnitus may be a sign of damage to your inner ear or the nerves that process hearing.

Out of 200 people who were surveyed, those who tended to use cellphones more over the previous four years had a higher risk of developing tinnitus. In fact, those who used cellphones for at least 10 minutes a day were nearly twice as likely to suffer from tinnitus. The theory is that the electromagnetic fields sent out by the phones may damage your brain's sound-processing structures.

If possible, use the speakerphone mode or a headset rather than listening and talking with the cellphone held right next to your ear. And limit your cell phone conversations when possible.

Along with using cellphones, listening to a portable digital music player, or MP3 player such as an iPod or other brand, may affect your hearing over time. Researchers tested five different brands of MP3 players, using several types of earphones or ear buds to see how much sound they put out. With the players set at top volume, all five brands produced more than 100 decibels of sound. Experts say you should avoid or limit the time you expose your ears to sounds this loud — equivalent to what you get at a rock concert or in a loud movie theater.

But that doesn't mean MP3 players are off-limits. Protect your hearing by taking these precautions as you listen to your tunes.

- Set a maximum volume limit on your player, around 50 percent or lower, so that no song will blast your ears.

117

- Invest in noise-canceling or noise-reduction earphones or ear buds that block background noise so you can keep the music volume low.

- Reduce the amount of time you spend listening to your music player.

Making a habit of using cotton swabs. Experts say you should not put anything in your ear that's smaller than the tip of your little finger. Cotton swabs may seem like the ideal tool to clean out earwax, but they may just push the wax further in. They can also puncture your eardrum. Instead, try this safe way to get wax — or almost anything — out of your ear fast.

Water irrigation, or a gentle warm water flush, can remove excess wax from your ears without harm. Here's how to do it yourself.

- Put a drop or two of warm mineral or vegetable oil in your ear, and wait about 15 minutes.

- Fill a bulb syringe with warm water, and gently flush your ear with it. Hold your head upright, then tilt to allow the water to drain out.

- Repeat the procedure a couple days later if you need to.

But don't put any liquid in your ear if you have punctured your eardrum.

You can ask your doctor for help irrigating your ears, but you'll save yourself the cost of a visit by doing it yourself. A study in England found that people who were taught how to irrigate their ears at home were less likely to come back to the doctor for the procedure later on.

Spending too much time in your little red convertible. When you drive or ride at 55 mph in a convertible with the top down, you subject your ears to sounds above 85 decibels. That's almost as loud as some lawn mowers, and loud enough to damage your hearing over time.

The risk is even greater if you turn up the radio while you ride in an effort to hear your music over the sound of the wind rushing by, researchers say.

To enjoy your roadster without losing your hearing, experts suggest these precautions.

- Keep your top-down driving off the highway, where you'll drive at lower speeds.

- Roll up the side windows when you put the car's top down.

- Wear earplugs.

Leaving the fruits and veggies on your plate. Eating carrots is good for your eyes, and it's also good for your ears. That's because vitamin A is a nutrient that can help protect against hearing loss.

Researchers in Australia followed nearly 3,000 people ages 50 years and older, keeping tabs on what they ate and whether they lost hearing over five years. Those who got the most vitamin A in their diets were 47 percent less likely to show moderate or severe hearing loss after five years than people who got the least vitamin A.

The lead researcher in the study explains that vitamin A protects auditory cells by blocking production of damaging free radicals in your body. Great sources of vitamin A include carrots, sweet potatoes, and pumpkin.

Other research has shown that older people with hearing loss also tend to have low blood levels of folic acid. Get the folic acid you need from lentils and chickpeas or greens like collards or turnip greens.

Easy ways to turn pet hassles into happiness

Your animal companion can keep you company at home, giving you someone to share meals and play with. He also provides reasons to get out and socialize, as you go for walks or head to the vet for a checkup. But owning a pet is a big responsibility, and sometimes a furry friend brings challenges in terms of keeping clean and staying safe. These simple tricks can help you live happily with your dog or cat.

Let your dog be your treadmill. Owning a dog is a great way to be sure you get some exercise. After all, most dogs really love a good, long walk.

Researchers in Michigan found that people who owned and walked their dogs were more likely to get the recommended amount of exercise than nonwalkers. About half the dog lovers got at least 30 minutes of exercise five or more times each week, while only one-third of those without dogs got that much.

And walking your dog seems to be an even better form of exercise than walking with a human friend. Fifty-four people in an assisted-living home were assigned to either walk five times a week or rest. Some of the walkers had a human friend join them, while the others were taken by bus to a local animal shelter, where they walked dogs.

After three months, people who walked the dogs were more consistent in getting their exercise than people who joined a human walking companion. The dogs were always eager to go for a walk, while human walkers sometimes helped each other find excuses for skipping the activity.

Results showed that people walking dogs greatly improved their fitness and increased their walking speeds during the study. Remarkably, some people actually stopped using canes and walkers.

If you do start walking, here's a way to get an extra fat-busting boost. Take a fish oil supplement right after your walk, and you can lower your cholesterol and lose more body fat.

One study found that taking fish oil capsules and walking 45 minutes three times a week each reduced body fat and improved heart risk factors in the people studied. But the combination of doing both worked even better over the 12 weeks of the study.

It really couldn't be easier. Aim for capsules containing 6 grams of fish oil daily to get the same amount of omega-3 fatty acids used in the research, and enjoy time on the trails with your favorite canine companion.

Why you should own a pet

Being an animal lover and owning a pet or two is not a sign you can't get along with people. Researchers found that people who own pets do better, socially speaking, than those who live in animal-free homes. Three studies showed various social benefits pets can provide to humans.

- Pet owners in one study were happier, healthier, and better adjusted socially than people without pets.

- People with dogs had greater feelings of self-esteem and feelings of belonging than people who didn't own a dog.

- Thinking about a favorite pet seemed to help young adults feel better after a difficult social experience.

Control fleas naturally. Turning to powerful chemical treatments to keep fleas off your pet can lead to short- and long-term health problems — even death. Veterinarians sometimes recommend flea shampoo with pyrethrin, an ingredient made from chrysanthemums, because it's safer than other insecticides. But even pyrethrin has some risks, so you may want to avoid it.

Instead, try a natural, nontoxic pet shampoo that works to keep fleas off your pet and out of your home. Look for one that contains the citrus oils d-limonene or linalool. These natural ingredients kill adult fleas and their eggs, and they'll leave your pet smelling citrus fresh. Brands like Adams d-Limonene Flea & Tick Shampoo are available at your veterinarian's office, grocery store, or online at retailers such as *www.amazon.com*.

Herbs like rosemary and lavender also have some flea-prevention effects. You can create an after-shampoo rinse to really make your pet smell great. Mix several drops each of rosemary oil, peppermint oil, tea tree oil, citronella oil, and eucalyptus oil in a cup of water. Shake it up and pour into a spray bottle to use on your pet.

If you're in a hurry, simply place a drop of flea-repelling rosemary or lavender oil on your dog's collar after he's dry from a bath.

Keep fur from flying. You've trimmed your dog's hair short, and you brush her daily when shedding season begins. There's one other trick to beat that shedding mess.

Run a vacuum attachment over your shedding dog, and pick up loose fur and excess dander before it can fly all over your house. Both Dyson and Bissell vacuum cleaner brands make attachments designed to whisk away pet hair from the source. Bissell even makes a model to fit other vacuum brands.

Some desperate pet owners even report using the regular hose attachment of their vacuum to clean up a furry friend, sometimes with holes drilled to reduce suction. Others recommend the machine's lighter "curtain" setting for the same reason. If your pet hates the noise of a vacuum, this trick may not work. But some pets actually enjoy being vacuumed.

Don't let your dog bring you down

Your pet may be a good friend, but he can also get you hurt.

Researchers at the Centers for Disease Control and Prevention (CDC) found that people older than 65 years are up to three times more likely than younger folks to end up in the emergency room after falling over their pets.

The report also brought to light injuries to owners who were pushed or pulled by their dogs, attacked by their cats, or tried to break up a fight between pets.

Take these precautions to avoid injury.

- Be aware of the risks of pet ownership, and consider whether you can handle a large dog or frisky puppy.

- Avoid risky behaviors like chasing a pet or walking an unruly dog.

- Place your pet's food and water bowls in a safe place on the floor, so you don't trip over them.

- Invest in obedience training for your dog.

Skip the costly cleanup products. It's bound to happen if you share your home with a dog or cat. Eventually, Fido or Fluffy will do their business on the carpet, leaving a smelly stain. But all you need is a common household item to clean and deodorize pet stains. White distilled vinegar is your go-to treatment that doesn't cost much and works like a dream.

First, test a hidden area of the carpet with vinegar to be sure it's colorfast. Then sprinkle some vinegar over the stain and wait a few minutes. Sponge the stain starting from the center and moving out, and blot with a dry cloth. Repeat if needed.

Vinegar also will repel your pet from that spot, possibly preventing him from marking in a favorite area again in the future. Both cats and dogs hate the smell of vinegar. They won't want to walk, sleep, or scratch in any area that smells like it.

6 terrific tricks to fend off loneliness

The average person has just two close confidants, usually people related to them, say researchers at Duke University. Even worse, 25 percent of people surveyed say they have no close relationships at all. Considering the physical and mental health risks of settling for a lonely life, it's worth the effort to be part of the gang. Try these simple methods to stop feeling lonely.

Get lost in a good book. Considering how much time many people spend reading fiction, it's not surprising they might feel a kind of emotional connection to the characters in books. And research shows it's true — you can feel a sense of belonging when you relate to fictional characters.

Forget the stereotype of the bookworm who turns to books for comfort because she can't handle real people. Studies have shown that people who read novels actually tend to be less socially isolated than those who read nonfiction or people who don't read at all. The explanation is simple. When you get into the mind of a fictional character and relate to their experiences, you are "practicing" your social skills. That makes you better able to empathize with real people in real relationships.

Researchers studied 195 seniors living in the Midwest about how they spent their time and whether they felt lonely. They found that people who do the most pleasure reading also reported the least loneliness. The only other activities that seemed to help were playing games and taking trips.

You can continue your lifelong habit of reading even while you give up other pursuits as you age. And when you wake up at night and your friends are still snoozing, turn to Sherlock Holmes, Jane Eyre, or Miss Jane Marple for company.

Meet up with your imaginary "friends" on TV. Just as you can feel connected to characters in a novel, you can also get comfort from your favorite television shows. Experts call this the social surrogacy hypothesis, or the idea that people turn to familiar characters in their favorite shows to get a sense of belonging.

And research shows it works. A set of four studies by psychologists found that people experienced greater feelings of belonging after tuning in to see their favorite shows — even after they were rejected by friends or relatives. Spending time, so to speak, with the characters they know also seemed to raise viewers' self-esteem.

So don't feel bad about needing to excuse yourself to watch your favorite show. You may be getting just the emotional boost you need.

Find sociable friends and keep them close. Spend time with people who are not lonely, and you may protect yourself from loneliness as well.

Harvard researchers looked at information from the Framingham Heart Study, which followed people in that Massachusetts town for more than 60 years. They discovered that loneliness tends to spread through a social network, kind of like a cold or other sickness.

Researcher John T. Cacioppo, Ph.D., explains how loneliness can spread. "We detected an extraordinary pattern of contagion that leads people to be moved to the edge of the social network when they become lonely," he said. "On the periphery, people have fewer friends, yet their loneliness leads them to losing the few ties they have left."

Overall, the researchers found that people tend to feel lonely an average of 48 days a year, but that number drops by two days a year for each friend you have. However, having just one lonely friend raises your risk of loneliness by up to 65 percent. The change was more striking among women than among men in the study.

Take comfort from the right foods. Smooth, creamy macaroni and cheese brings back happy childhood memories, and that bowl of chicken noodle soup makes you think of the warmth of home. So it makes sense that eating your favorite comfort foods can ease loneliness.

Researchers had people do a brief writing project about a fight with someone close to them, assessing their feelings of loneliness. Then they wrote about either a favorite comfort food or a new food. Loneliness was measured again. People who had recalled a comfort food felt less lonely afterward.

126

"We have found that comfort foods are foods which are consistently associated with those close to us," says study author Jordan Troisi, a graduate student at the University of Buffalo. "Thinking about or consuming these foods later then serves as a reminder of those close others."

The researchers also did a second experiment, allowing people to eat chicken soup in the lab. Then they were tested to see how much they were thinking about relationships. People who considered chicken soup to be a "comfort food" had more thoughts about people they cared for than those with more neutral thoughts about chicken soup.

You'll need to identify your personal comfort food to know what to eat to feel closer to those you love.

Join others to get active. Sometimes you just need to make a small effort to be social and spend time with other people. Get out of the house and meet with others at church or a community center, or call an old friend to have lunch together.

Besides making you happier, being social can also affect your weight. A study on mice found that those living in social situations as opposed to isolation lost white fat and gained brown fat — the energy-burning type. That helped the mice lose weight, just by living in a group.

Kill two birds with one stone by doing group exercise. It's old news that you can find an exercise group for yoga, aerobics, tai chi, or line dancing, saving you money over the cost of a personal trainer. But did you know you can also find a group to get involved in more solo pursuits like cycling, running, speed walking, hiking, and swimming? Look for group exercise opportunities at your local senior center, park and recreation facility, church, YMCA, or community college.

For a group workout without going outside, connect over an active video game like Nintendo Wii tennis or Xbox Kinect bowling. Research shows you can raise your heart rate when you play these active electronic games, plus you'll need a group to get the full effect of competition. Some senior centers already have active game systems available.

Change the way you think. When writer Henry David Thoreau built his tiny home on the shores of Walden Pond, he was looking for a solitary existence that would let him be alone with his thoughts. "I love to be alone," Thoreau wrote. "I never found the companion that was so companionable as solitude. We are for the most part more lonely when we go abroad among men than when we stay in our chambers."

Like Thoreau, you can enjoy the blessings of time alone if you decide you want to. But if you do want to have more — and better — relationships, you may need to work on yourself first.

Researchers looked back at some previous studies to figure out which treatment for loneliness seemed to work best. They found that using cognitive behavioral therapy (CBT) to help people change their thoughts worked better than three other key methods:

- improving social skills

- enhancing social support

- finding new opportunities for social contact

CBT can be helpful in dealing with depression, eating disorders, and other problems, but in this instance it helped people change the way they think about handling other people and being in social situations. To put it simply, people learned to squelch that little voice in their heads that makes them hesitate to deal with others. They learned to avoid the vicious cycle of negative thoughts and tendency to become isolated. In this case, the problem really was all in their heads.

Avoid health risks of a solitary life

Stay connected to other people, and you ward off loneliness. Isolate yourself, and you face real health risks. Experts say staying connected can cut your risk of death over time by up to 50 percent. But isolation can be as deadly as smoking or being overweight.

- Your blood pressure rises faster as you age. In one study, the loneliest people saw a systolic blood pressure rise of 14.4 mmHg more over four years than in socially connected folks.

- You may gain weight. Mice in a study lost weight when they lived in a social situation rather than in isolation.

- Eating right may be a thing of the past. Seniors who live alone tend to spend less time preparing and eating healthy meals.

- Your immune system gets out of whack, causing stress and putting you at risk of infections, cancer, and heart disease.

Best ways to beat fatigue and boost energy

Quick pick-me-ups to beat the afternoon slump

Your mind keeps drifting, your head droops drowsily, and every attempt to move or concentrate feels like swimming upstream through thick, sweet molasses. Before you surrender to the Sandman, re-energize with one of these pick-me-ups.

Enjoy the world's most perfect snack. It's full of fiber, vitamins, potassium, and magnesium and a favorite energy source of endurance athletes.

What is it? It's the humble banana — and it revitalizes you with two kinds of energy-building fuel. The simple sugars in the banana give you an instant lift, but that energy doesn't vanish minutes later in a dramatic sugar crash. Instead, you get sustained energy because the banana has fiber that slows your body's ability to absorb simple sugars. That means you continue receiving little bursts of energy long after the banana is gone.

In fact, a recent study of cyclists participating in a 75-kilometer (47-mile) time trial found that those who ate bananas boosted their performance just as much as cyclists who guzzled sports drinks.

As if that's not enough, bananas can help your body fight cancer, heart disease, insomnia, and more. The best part — one small to medium banana only averages 100 calories, so you can gain energy without gaining weight.

Unwrap a mini-treat. Research shows chewing gum can make you more alert. Gum may even improve your thinking ability, one study suggests. Sugarless gum is the best choice for your teeth, but that doesn't mean it can't taste good. Read on to find out why minty or cinnamon-flavored gum may be your best bet.

Sniff a fragrance. The afternoon slump can feel remarkably similar to that tired, sluggish feeling you get after driving for hours. Fortunately, a West Virginia study found that people who drove a long time felt more alert when the scent of cinnamon or peppermint was in the air. Likewise, a Japanese study discovered the scent of lemon helped people pep up. Aromas like rosemary or eucalyptus may help revive you, too.

You can easily experiment with these scents to see what works best for you. For example, chew cinnamon or mint gum, pop a breath mint, place a few eucalyptus branches in a vase, drink peppermint or rosemary tea, or enjoy a lemon-scented or cinnamon-scented tea.

Press key points. Try the ancient art of Chinese acupressure to renew your energy. A small University of Michigan study found that the acupressure point at the center of the top of your head was a key part of a successful re-energizing strategy. Tap that point with your fingers for three minutes to help you recharge. You can also try massaging the webbed area between your big toe and second toe — another acupressure point. Massage that area for several minutes, and you may find yourself feeling more energetic.

Copy your cat. Stop and stretch just like a cat would, or stretch in whatever way rejuvenates you the most. Stretching makes you breathe more deeply, so you send more oxygen to your drowsy brain. Stretching after a period of stillness also releases tension in your muscles. For extra energizing power, try this "ancient Chinese secret." While seated on the floor with your legs straight out in front of you, bend forward, reach out, and try to touch your toes without rounding your back. This action reportedly helps release energy from your lower back area.

Step into the sunshine. Brighten your day for a few minutes, and you may be surprised at how much livelier you feel. Research shows that bright light causes changes in your brain that make you more alert. In fact, just 21 minutes of bright white light was enough to create changes in the brain scans of Belgian study participants. So just a few minutes outside in the sunlight or basking by a sunny window may be all you need.

Turn on a toe-tapper. Pull out your MP3 or CD player or turn on the radio, and look for an energetic tune that will get your feet tapping and your blood pumping. If you have a computer, you can search for an old favorite song at *www.youtube.com*. Even listening to just one song may be enough to wake you up and chase the doldrums away.

Pour yourself a tall one. Fatigue is one of the first signs your body is running low on water. In fact, you only need to lose 2 percent of your body's water weight to be mildly dehydrated. If you've been exerting yourself in hot weather, or you've had little to drink during the last few hours, drink some water to replenish your energy and improve your concentration.

5 things you should know about energy drinks

Some energy drinks and energy shots may contain much more caffeine than you expect if guarana is in the ingredient list. Just 1 milligram (mg) of guarana may contain up to 80 mg of caffeine, but manufacturers are not required to include this amount in the caffeine content on the label. Here are four more surprising facts.

- The amount of caffeine listed on an energy drink's label may only be for one serving, but a single can may contain two or more servings.

- Some energy drinks have up to 14 times more caffeine than a single can of Coca-Cola.

- One 5-hour ENERGY shot contains more than 200 mg of caffeine, and another brand of energy shot contains 500 mg per serving.

- The caffeine in energy drinks and energy shots may interact with some medications.

Spread out your calories. To help prevent tomorrow's afternoon slump, plan to eat five or six small meals or large snacks throughout the day. As a result, your energy will no longer spike after meals and quickly vanish. Instead, you will get smaller bursts of energy all day long.

For best results, avoid snacks that only contain sugary or starchy foods with no fiber. Cookies, snack cakes, and potato chips may give you an instant lift, but that energy fades quickly. For energy that sticks with you, include foods with fiber, lean protein, or a little healthy fat in both your small meals and your large snacks.

This may seem easier to do in meals than in snacks, so here's a little help to get started. Good snack choices include hearty whole grains, a handful of nuts, fruit with low-fat cheese, fruit and nut combinations, tuna on whole-grain crackers, apple slices painted with peanut butter, blueberries mixed into nonfat yogurt, vegetables dipped in hummus, or whole-grain toast with peanut butter.

3 secrets for lasting energy

A quick pick-me-up is fine for the occasional afternoon slump, but you want energy that lasts. To get it, make your lifestyle and diet as healthy as possible, and consider boosting your energy levels with one of these strategies.

Try a fatigue-fighting herb. During their treatment, most cancer patients struggle with an utterly draining fatigue that doesn't respond to treatment. But research suggests the herb ginseng may make a difference — and if it can work for cancer patients, it could work for you, too.

Two Mayo Clinic studies of cancer patients put ginseng to the test. In the most recent one, all participants filled out questionnaires that helped rate how fatigued they were. For the next eight weeks, half the participants took 2,000 milligrams (mg) of ginseng daily, while the other half took placebo capsules. Both groups reported less exhaustion by the end of the eight weeks, but the ginseng group reported twice as much improvement as the placebo group.

Keep in mind these results are considered preliminary because they have only been presented at a medical conference. Research is not considered fully reliable until independent scientists have examined the study and declared it accurate enough to be published in an academic journal.

Talk to your doctor before you try ginseng. This herb is not safe for everyone. Capsules made from ginseng extract instead of pure ground ginseng are dangerous for people who have breast cancer. But if your doctor gives you the green light, remember that several different types of ginseng are available. Look for *Panax quinquefolius* on the label if you want the same energizing ginseng used in the study.

> ## *Hidden risks of supplements*
>
> Supplements are not regulated or checked by the Food and Drug Administration (FDA.) That means some may not contain the ingredients on their labels, and some may even contain contaminants.
>
> To avoid these problems, look for supplements that display the National Sanitation Foundation (NSF) or U.S. Pharmacopeial Convention (USP) seal of approval on their labels.
>
> These seals guarantee the product has passed tests for purity and accurate product labeling. Visit *www.usp.org or www.nsf.org* for supplements that have passed this testing.

Increase your pep. Imagine a miracle drug that could rev up your endurance in as little as seven days. Two recent studies suggest quercetin can do just that, but it's not a drug. It's a natural compound in foods and supplements. Recent animal and human studies show that "natural" doesn't mean it's not powerful.

A University of South Carolina study found that mice fed quercetin for seven days not only increased their endurance, but also the amount of time they voluntarily spent running on a wheel. According to the researchers, this happened because quercetin causes mitochondria in your brain and muscles to multiply.

Mitochondria are like tiny power plants in your cells that provide you with energy. The researchers think the extra supply of mitochondria could be one reason why the mice ran more. But the scientists also point out that quercetin may help block a compound called adenosine from connecting to adenosine receptors in your brain. As a result, quercetin may have a mild stimulant effect that helps increase both the desire and the energy to exercise.

But quercetin doesn't just work in mice. A small study found that college students also increased their endurance after just seven days of taking 1,000 mg of quercetin daily.

To try quercetin for yourself, start with revitalizing foods rich in this nutrient. That includes greens like radicchio, rocket, or kale; cooked onions; asparagus; and cranberries. The quercetin in these foods ranges from almost 15 mg in a 3-ounce portion to 66 mg.

If you can't get enough quercetin from food, ask your doctor if you can safely take supplements. Quercetin is generally considered safe, but cases of kidney damage have been reported in a few people who took more than 1,000 mg a day, and side effects like headaches or upset stomach sometimes occur at lower doses.

On the other hand, if your doctor approves quercetin for you, you may be in for a pleasant surprise. Quercetin supplements have been clinically proven to protect brain cells, block cholesterol buildup, prevent ulcers, fight cancer and lung disease, and relieve allergies.

Help your body create energy. You may not think of zinc as an energy booster, but people who don't get enough of this amazing mineral have less strength and tire more quickly. This may happen because your body depends on zinc-containing enzymes for many energy-related processes — including the ones that control muscle energy.

When you use your muscles, waste products like carbon dioxide build up inside them. If too much carbon dioxide piles up, your muscles become fatigued. Fortunately, a zinc-containing enzyme called carbonic anhydrase helps rush carbon dioxide away from your muscles so you can keep your energy up. But if you don't get enough zinc, carbonic anhydrase can't do its job. That may be why research has linked low zinc levels to a drop in energy — even while you are at rest.

To make sure you get enough zinc to help fend off fatigue, eat a variety of these easy-to-find foods that can give you all the zinc you need.

- a one-cup serving of Product 19 or Wheaties cereal

- a one-cup serving of trail mix with chocolate chips, salted nuts, and seeds

- a one-cup serving of canned baked beans with pork and tomato sauce

- a 3-ounce serving of lean beef steak or ground beef

- a one-cup serving of canned blue crab or roasted turkey

- one fast food chimichanga with beef

Making sure you take in enough zinc may also have other rewards. Zinc also helps fight free radicals, heal wounds, prevent infections, fight macular degeneration, and sharpen your sense of taste.

4 snooze-inducers to watch out for

No matter how early you go to bed, you're still exhausted all the time, and you can't imagine why. Fortunately, you don't need Sherlock Holmes or Jane Marple to help you find out. If you've crossed off all the usual suspects, check for these four unexpected problems that could determine whether you feel fatigued or fantastic.

Lack of vitamin B12. Up to 15 percent of older adults are deficient in this important B vitamin because they no longer have enough stomach acid to help absorb the natural form of B12 from food. You may also be low in this vitamin if one of these describes you.

- You eat a restricted diet.

- You regularly take acid-reducing drugs like omeprazole (Prilosec, Zegerid), lansoprazole (Prevacid), cimetidine (Tagamet), ranitidine (Zantac), or famotidine (Pepcid).

- You take the diabetes drug Metformin.

- You have a condition, like celiac disease, that prevents you from absorbing nutrients well.

Knowing your risk of B12 deficiency is important because constant fatigue is one sign you may be low on this vitamin. Other possible symptoms include appetite loss, sore tongue, constipation, anemia, weight loss, weakness, and balance problems. You may also experience brain- or nerve-related symptoms like memory loss, difficulty walking, numbness or tingling in your arms or legs, depression, disorientation, and dementia.

Even worse, if you are deficient for too long, adding more B12 may come too late to undo nerve- and brain-related damage. Fortunately, reversing low B12 levels can be easy, and it may bring unexpected rewards.

For example, low B12 levels have been linked to frailty in older adults. So if you want to stay active and vigorous well into your senior years, be sure to get enough of this important vitamin. It will help you have more energy and feel healthier, and as a bonus, you'll get stronger hair and nails.

To find out whether you have a B12 deficiency, talk to your doctor. She can test your levels and prescribe injections or recommend supplements if you need them. Meanwhile, eat cereals and other foods fortified with B12. People who don't have enough stomach acid to absorb natural B12 can still absorb some of the synthetic B12 in fortified foods and supplements.

Beware of drugs that sap your energy

Statins are not the only drugs that may cause fatigue. Consider this list of common offenders.

- prescription painkillers
- steroids
- colchicine
- heart medications
- high blood pressure drugs including diuretics
- cholesterol-lowering drugs including fenofibrates
- anti-anxiety drugs, tranquilizers, and antidepressants
- tetracycline and other antibiotics
- over-the-counter and prescription allergy or cold medications that contain antihistamines like diphenhydramine

If you suspect one of your prescription medications is sapping your energy, don't stop taking it without your doctor's permission. That can be dangerous. Check *www.drugs.com*, or ask your pharmacist if fatigue is a side effect of your prescription.

If so, talk to your doctor. She can lower your dosage, switch to another medication, eliminate the drug, or suggest another change to relieve your fatigue.

Side effects of common drugs. Statins are great for lowering cholesterol, but if you've been feeling tired lately, they could be the problem, a new study suggests. After six months of taking a low-dose statin, 40 percent of women participating in the study reported more fatigue during exercise or lower energy levels all the time. Statin drugs include atorvastatin (Lipitor), fluvastatin (Lescol), rosuvastatin (Crestor), lovastatin (Mevacor), pravastatin (Pravachol), and simvastatin (Zocor).

Drug side effects like fatigue may begin when you start a new medication, but they can also appear when you switch to a new brand of the same drug, when your doctor raises the dosage, or even after you have taken a drug for a while. See the box "Beware of drugs that sap your energy" to see what other meds could be tiring you out.

Out-of-whack thyroid gland. Constant weariness may mean one of your body's energy managers is acting up. The thyroid gland inside your neck produces thyroid hormone, which helps manage your body's energy. The thyroid is more likely to be the cause of your fatigue if other members of your family have had thyroid problems, too.

Oddly enough, fatigue can be a symptom of a thyroid gland that produces too little thyroid hormone (hypothyroidism,) but it can also occur if your thyroid produces too much of the hormone (hyperthyroidism). Your other symptoms may help you tell which one may be your problem.

- Hypothyroidism (underactive thyroid) — weight gain, lack of energy, weakness, depression, memory problems, dry and itchy skin, high sensitivity to cold, daytime sleepiness, coarse and thinning hair, brittle hair or nails, or a yellow or orange tint in your skin.

- Hyperthyroidism (overactive thyroid) — weight loss, high sensitivity to heat, hand tremors, difficulty sleeping, sweating, increased heart rate, irritability, anxiety, muscle weakness, or enlarged thyroid.

You may not have all of these symptoms. In fact, older adults often develop only one or two symptoms. Fortunately, your doctor can order blood tests to find out whether your thyroid is underactive, overactive, or just right.

Constant rush of adrenaline. Think about the last time you had a thrilling day planned. When the day arrived, you were probably so excited that you experienced an adrenaline rush. That made your heart pound and kept your energy high. After the excitement ended and the adrenaline rush wore off, you may have been surprised by how tired you suddenly were.

Surprising source of fatigue

Pain and fatigue? It may not be arthritis or fibromyalgia after all. Ask your doctor to check for a more common — and treatable — ailment instead.

Two recent reviews of research suggest that fatigue and body pain may be symptoms of chronic rhinosinusitis (CRS), a condition where your nasal sinuses are constantly inflamed, swollen, and often cause facial pain or hay fever symptoms. Scientists found that people with CRS who reported fatigue or body pain saw those symptoms improve after undergoing endoscopic sinus surgery.

Earlier studies have also linked fatigue and body pain with CRS. So ask your doctor if chronic sinus troubles could be your problem. CRS medications or surgery just may give you the relief you've been waiting for.

Stress works nearly the same way. Your body releases adrenaline to give you energy to cope with the cause of your stress. If the stress ends quickly, you may realize you're tired and rest to recover. But if the stress is continuous, the adrenaline keeps coming, and you keep burning up your body's energy by the truckload. Naturally, this contributes to physical and mental exhaustion, and may cause fatigue.

If you're not sure whether stress is stealing your energy, put it to the test. Practice stress management exercises every day, and see if you feel more energetic. For example, take 10 minutes for a mental vacation at the beach or your favorite mountain spot. Imagine in vivid detail each of the sights, sounds, smells, and activities you would experience if you were spending a day there.

For more stress management exercises, see "6 serene secrets to soothing stress" in the *Top tips for tension prevention* chapter.

Lock sleep thieves away for good

You have counted sheep so many times that the sheep are threatening to go on strike — or maybe you sleep the night through but wake up exhausted. If this describes you, a little detective work may help you nab your sleep thief and put this "repeat offender" away for life.

Reverse the call of nature. Always hurrying to the bathroom? One simple dietary change could end persistent incontinence. Stop eating and drinking things that irritate your bladder. For example, cut out acidic drinks like tomato juice, orange juice, other citrus juices, and even cranberry juice. While cranberry juice may help if you have a urinary tract infection, it irritates your bladder and makes things worse if you have incontinence or an overactive bladder.

Replace acidic drinks with apple juice, grape juice, cherry juice, and water. But remember, acidic drinks are not the only things that may irritate your bladder, so temporarily stop drinking and eating the following items, too.

- caffeinated foods and beverages including decaffeinated coffee and tea, plus high caffeine medications like Excedrin

- carbonated drinks including caffeine-free versions

- alcoholic beverages

- chocolate, hot chocolate

- milk including chocolate milk

- drinks and foods with sugar, honey, corn syrup, or artificial sweeteners

- spicy foods

Temporarily eliminate all these from your diet for three weeks, and see if you make fewer trips to the bathroom at night. After that three weeks, add back just one category of food or beverage during each of the following weeks. For example, you might add back spicy foods the first week. If your symptoms return that week, you must avoid that food category from now on, and you may want to wait a week before adding back any other foods or drinks. If your missing symptoms stay gone, you can keep eating or drinking the items in that category.

Sound suggestions for a good night's sleep

If you don't know what's causing your sleeplessness, make sure you practice good stress management, limit your caffeine to the first half of the day, and limit alcohol. Next, ask your doctor for information on good sleep hygiene, or visit *www.bedroom.sleepfoundation.org* on the Internet for details on improving your sleep environment and sleep-affecting habits.

Search for allergens in your bedroom. On a beautiful spring day, you could throw open your bedroom windows or even play with your pet outside. But those choices may cause allergy symptoms that night if you're allergic to pollens, pets, or dust mites. Fortunately, it's easy to beat allergies in your bedroom so you can breathe easier when you sleep.

To start, leave the bedroom windows closed so the wind can't blow pollen inside and deposit it on your bedding, furniture, and carpet. In addition, don't let your pet sleep or spend time in your bedroom. Rover or Fluffy may leave pet dander or pollen behind.

Pollen can also deposit itself in your clothes, hair, and skin while you are outdoors. Don't take it with you to bed. Instead shower, shampoo, and use a nasal rinse before sleeping. But even with these precautions, some pollen, pet dander, or dust mites may still reach your bedding, so wash it all, including pillows, once a week in water over 150 degrees.

Relieve stuffy nose and sinuses. Congestion and sinus problems making you miserable? Stop sinus stuffiness with one very cheap, safe remedy — nasal irrigation. This procedure gently rinses your nasal passages to get rid of any viruses, bacteria, pollen, allergens, dust, or mucus lurking there. Experts and studies suggest this may work better than expensive drugs and sprays.

In fact, two studies found that people who use nasal irrigation need fewer antibiotics or nasal sprays than people who don't. Study participants who used nasal irrigation also reported fewer and less severe symptoms. What's more, a new review of research by the Infectious Diseases Society of America recommends nasal irrigation to adults with chronic sinus problems. To try nasal irrigation, you will need:

- a neti pot or bulb syringe. The neti pot resembles Aladdin's magic lamp or a teapot, and the bulb syringe features a squeezable bulb at one end and a hollow tube at the other. Both products are available at drugstores.

- distilled water or boiled water. Don't use tap water unless you have boiled it for one to three minutes and let it cool. Unboiled tap water may contain *Naegleria fowleri*, a microbe that is harmless if you drink it but can cause brain infection and death if it enters your nose.

- salt. The American Academy of Allergy, Asthma, and Immunology recommends canning or pickling salt because table salt may contain anti-caking agents or other additives that may irritate nasal passages. If you must use table salt, only use the noniodized kind.

- baking soda. This buffers the salt to soothe your sinuses.

To put these ingredients to work, mix one-half teaspoon of salt and one-quarter teaspoon of baking soda into 8 ounces of water. Pour it into the neti pot, or suction the water into the bulb syringe. Tilt your head sideways over a sink, and slowly pour or squeeze the mixture into one nostril so it runs out the other nostril. Use up half the mixture. Turn your head to the other side, and pour the remaining mixture into the other nostril. Gently blow your nose after the water has drained out.

Nasal irrigation may not be for everyone. One study suggests that some people have fewer sinus infections when they don't use nasal irrigation every day. If you feel long-term nasal irrigation has made your symptoms worse, follow the advice of the study's lead researcher. Only use nasal irrigation for short periods of time when you are experiencing symptoms.

Calm your restless legs. Every time you get still, that crawling or tingling in your legs sets in, and you must move them to ease the discomfort. This may be a symptom of Restless Leg

Syndrome (RLS), and it can interfere with your sleep. If you have this symptom, ask your doctor whether you could have RLS and iron deficiency. If you have these problems, she can prescribe iron supplements and other helpful treatments.

Meanwhile, start taking smart steps to ease your symptoms. Get regular exercise, and make sure you get enough iron in your diet. Good sources of this essential mineral include Product 19 cereal, fortified oatmeal, clams, beef, poultry, and canned baked beans with pork and tomato sauce.

Swap drugs for cherries. If your insomnia continues in spite of these changes, don't buy any sleep aids just yet. Sleeping pills are not only addictive, they may also have dangerous side effects like sleep driving, high blood pressure, confusion, and temporary memory loss. They can also cause sleepwalking, sleep binge-eating, headaches, constipation, dizziness, weakness, nausea, morning-after grogginess, and, sometimes, rebound insomnia that makes the original insomnia seem mild.

For a good night's sleep, pass up the sleeping pills, and snack on melatonin-rich cherry juice or cherries instead. Two small studies suggest cherry juice can be highly effective in helping you sleep. An American study discovered that drinking Montmorency tart cherry juice twice a day helped people spend less time awake during the night. But drinking a more concentrated version of tart cherry juice twice a day led to getting more sleep and sounder sleep, a British study reported.

The study also revealed that the juice boosted melatonin levels. This is important because melatonin affects your body temperature in a way that helps you sleep. Cherries also contain antioxidants and anti-inflammatory compounds that may promote sleep. If you try cherries, remember these tips.

- The study participants drank Montmorency tart cherry juice, but experts say you can eat dried, frozen, or fresh versions of these cherries instead. Start with a handful of fresh or dried cherries, and add cherries or switch to juice if you need more.

- Eat or drink your cherries once during early morning and again two to three hours before bedtime.

If your sleep problems persist in spite of several weeks of cherries, medications or health conditions like sleep apnea may be contributing to your insomnia. See your doctor to find out.

Slip into slumber naturally

Restful nights can be yours again with valerian. Studies suggest this popular herb can help ease you into dreamland, so you get to sleep faster and sleep better.

Valerian not only contains compounds that make you feel sleepy but also valeric acid to help release the relaxing compound gamma-aminobutyric acid. Even better, valerian is not habit-forming and doesn't leave you with a groggy, sluggish feeling the next morning. Experts recommend 300 to 600 milligrams standardized to a 1-percent valerenic acid dose. Take it an hour before bed every night, and you should begin seeing results within a few weeks.

But before you buy valerian, ask your doctor if the herb is safe for you. Valerian may interact with prescription or over-the-counter medications you take, and it may cause insomnia if taken for longer than three months.

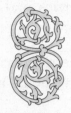

Natural, low-cost secrets to a healthy home

Scrub your house without lifting a finger

Forget the elbow grease. Nobody wants to work hard to clean things around the house. Save your energy for the golf course, and try these tricks to get the cleaning done without breaking a sweat.

Give your dishwasher an extra chore. Don't tackle the greasy job of cleaning your oven and stove fans and filters by hand. Remove these items from their housings, and place in the top rack of the dishwasher. Run them through a full wash cycle, and see how clean they get with no scrubbing.

You can also use your dishwasher to clean other items from all around your house.

- Kitchen sponge. Toss it in the closed part of the utensil basket, and sanitize your sponge on the hottest wash cycle.

- Costume jewelry. Tie up dull chains and rings in a pair of pantyhose, then secure to the top rack with a bread tie. They'll come out looking shiny and new.

- Glass domes from light fixtures. Unless these are painted and delicate, you can wash them in the top rack.

- Vent covers. Never again will you cut your fingers dusting the tiny slats of unpainted steel, aluminum, or plastic covers.

- Soap dishes from the bathroom, kitchen, or mud room.

Let the crock clean itself. Making dinner in a slow cooker is easy and hands-off. But — especially if the ceramic pot doesn't lift out of its electrical base — cleanup can be a real pain.

Here's how to get the job done with no scrubbing. Fill the slow cooker with water to just above the line of crustiness. Turn it on low, and let the heat and water soften up the mess. After about 20 minutes, turn off and unplug the cooker, then empty out the water. You'll be able to wipe away the mess with a sponge. Be careful not to burn your fingers.

A similar no-fuss trick removes mineral stains from a crock. Fill it three-quarters with hot water and a cup of white vinegar. Cover and cook on high power for two hours. Then clean as usual.

Tell mites to be gone. House dust mites can trigger allergies in some people, plus they're just downright gross. Spending

149

$80 to clean your mattress of these ugly critters doesn't make sense when there's a no-cost, no-chemical treatment you can do yourself.

It's as simple as placing mite-infested items like pillows, blankets, and mattresses outside in the sunlight on a hot summer day. Researchers found they could kill 100 percent of both adult mites and their eggs by exposing them to dry heat for a few hours. It might take as long as five hours to take care of them all, and it's best to wait for a sunny summer day when temperatures are as high as possible — even above 95 degrees Fahrenheit.

If you don't live where the weather gets this hot, try washing sheets in hot water instead of warm. Researchers found a water temperature of 140 degrees Fahrenheit killed mites in infested linens, while a warm setting of 104 degrees didn't work as well.

Turn your microwave into a self-cleaning oven. Leave a bowl of spaghetti in the microwave too long, and you may hear it go "boom." Don't look now, but you get to clean up tomato sauce from the ceiling and walls of the appliance.

If you've avoided this icky job for too long, try this trick to soften the crusty mess so it wipes away easily. Put a vinegar-water mixture in a medium-sized bowl, and place it in the microwave. Heat the mixture for five minutes, then wipe. No scrubbing required.

Bring power to the project. Electric toothbrushes let you clean between your teeth easily. They can also help clean hard-to-reach places in your house.

Use an inexpensive battery-powered toothbrush to clean those cracks and crevices, like around the sink faucets, in tile grout, and in corners of the baseboards. Just sprinkle powdered cleanser, or spray on a household cleaner, and let the brush do the work.

You can find cheap electric toothbrushes for $5 or $10 at your grocery store or online at sites like *www.amazon.com*. Look for Crest Spinbrush or Oral-B Pulsar.

Blow out pet hair. Toss your dog's bed cover into the dryer for 10 minutes, and let the machine remove fur buildup. It will be collected for you in the dryer's lint trap for easy removal. Clean the lint trap immediately to avoid starting a fire and to keep your dryer running efficiently.

If the bed cover can't be removed, use a sticky lint roller to collect the dog hair. Or make your own by spritzing some hairspray onto a clean cloth. The fur will be attracted to the cloth for easy cleaning.

Don't break the bank on mite solutions

You can pay $10,000 for a vacuum cleaner marketed to clear up asthma by removing mite allergens from your home. Don't do it. Experts say even the most expensive and specialized mite-control tools and techniques probably won't solve your problem.

Researchers looked at 54 studies on mite-control measures to see if they helped some 3,000 people with asthma made worse by mite allergens. Overall, the asthma sufferers didn't benefit, meaning their breathing did not improve and they used just as much medication.

It may sound strange, but experts say even if you remove nearly all mites from your home, the few that remain may still cause problems. And if you're sensitive to mites, you're probably also bothered by other allergens.

Clean for pennies with 6 simple products

Count the bottles of cleaning solutions under your kitchen sink, in your laundry room, and on that extra shelf in your bathroom. Then multiply that number by $4 or $5, and consider what you could have done with that money instead. Simplify your cleaning routine by using cheap and natural solutions, and get rid of those unused cleaning products. These are the only six cleaning products you need.

Baking soda is the powerhouse in your pantry. This household wonder cleaner is a mild abrasive, so it can scour pots, pans, sinks, bathtubs, and ovens without scratching. You can also use it on countertops, tile, glass, and walls. Mix it with hydrogen peroxide for a grout cleaner, or sprinkle it in your toilet for a daily cleansing.

Just like you prevent bad smells in your refrigerator with an open box of baking soda, you can use it to keep your bathroom smelling fresh. Leave out a small dish of baking soda on the counter to absorb odors.

Vinegar cuts through grease. That 5 percent acetic acid in household vinegar lets it whisk away a greasy mess. But never use vinegar to clean marble in your home, since it can react with the marble and create pitting.

Here's how to use white vinegar to clean walls and wood floors. Mix one cup vinegar into a gallon of hot water, adding a tablespoon of lemon oil if you like. Use a damp rag or mop to wipe down sticky walls or clean a grimy floor, leaving no residue.

Lemon juice cleans like a charm. Use this natural acidic wonder to polish metal, cut grease, and lighten laundry stains. Mix it with water for an inexpensive glass cleaner.

You can also make a fresh-smelling cleaning solution from citrus peels. Save rinds from oranges, lemons, limes, or grapefruit, and put them in a jar of white vinegar. Seal the jar, and let brew for four weeks. Strain the liquid, and use your citrus solution to clean just like regular vinegar. It's super cheap and easy.

Fix bleach splatter fast

Don't toss out your favorite top or slacks with a bleach splatter. Use a waterproof permanent marker — like Sharpie or Pigma pens — to add color back into the fabric where bleach has caused fading. Markers come in dozens of shades, so it's likely you'll find one to match your garment.

Liquid dish soap lets you clean gently. It works on dishes, and it's also great to clean all around your house. Make your own soft scrub by mixing a cup of baking soda with warm water and a few drops of liquid soap. Use just enough water to form a paste, and mix only what you need so it won't dry out.

Apply this mixture to enamel or porcelain, then let it set for a few minutes. You'll have no trouble wiping away the mess.

Bleach kills germs everywhere. "Cleaning" refers to removing dirt, while "sanitizing" or "disinfecting" means killing 99 to 100 percent of germs. Bleach kills the bacteria that can cause food poisoning, so it's a great tool in the kitchen.

Food safety specialist Lydia Medeiros tested using diluted bleach to kill bacteria on countertops, cutting boards, utensils, and dishes. Her team found that a scant teaspoon of bleach mixed into a quart of water killed more than 99 percent of dangerous bacteria in just one minute.

"Not many things will kill *E. coli* at room temperature, and this did," Medeiros said.

Use bleach safely by wearing gloves and keeping the area ventilated. Also, never mix bleach with ammonia or toilet bowl cleaner, since it can produce dangerous fumes.

Borax does great things outside the laundry. This inexpensive laundry booster can work in place of bleach, wiping out germs and keeping your family healthy.

Borax, a natural mineral, kills mold wherever it's found. Just mix one-half cup borax into a gallon of hot water, and wipe down surfaces prone to that black crud.

Make your own air freshener

Save money while you fill your rooms with the scent you choose. Soak a cotton ball with your favorite cologne and place in a glass jar without a lid. When the fragrance starts to fade, replace the cotton ball with a fresh one.

8 dangerous kitchen habits to avoid

The kitchen should be the heart of your home, so the last thing you want to do is harm your family by what goes on there. Food poisoning can be spread in foods served at restaurants or cafeterias, but sometimes it happens in your own kitchen. Keep your family safe by steering clear of these eight kitchen habits that can make you sick.

Using unclean grocery bags. Only 15 percent of Americans regularly wash those eco-friendly reusable grocery bags. But leaking milk or spilled meat juices can contaminate the bags with disease-causing microbes, such as *salmonella, listeria,* or *E. coli.* The foodborne diseases these cause can lead to kidney failure, chronic arthritis, brain or nerve damage, and even death.

"Unwashed grocery bags are lingering with bacteria which can easily contaminate your foods," warns Ruth Frechman, registered dietitian and spokesperson for the Academy of Nutrition and Dietetics. "Cross-contamination occurs when juices from raw meats or germs from unclean objects come in contact with cooked or ready-to-eat foods like breads or produce."

But you can stop the spread of disease and still get lots of uses from your reusable bags.

"Food poisoning can easily be prevented with practical steps, such as cleaning grocery totes and separating raw meats from ready-to-eat foods when shopping, cooking, serving, and storing foods," Frechman says.

Wash bags often with hot, soapy water, either in the washing machine or in the sink. And don't place bags on a dirty kitchen counter.

Skipping "stand" time for microwavable meals. You assume your frozen lunch is already cooked, but what you don't know about frozen convenience meals could make you sick — or even kill you. The Food and Drug Administration warns that one in six Americans will become ill from food poisoning this year.

It also points out that stand time is an important part of the cooking process, since this extra time lets heat be conducted all the way to the center of the food. So if your frozen lasagna says, "Cook in microwave for four minutes, let stand for two minutes," follow it to the letter. Then you'll know the food is cooked properly, killing harmful bacteria.

Storing deli meat in the store package. Dangerous bacteria like *listeria* can have a field day in a deli, jumping from the meat slicer to the scale to the bag your meat is placed in. Keep the danger to a minimum by putting your purchase in a fresh bag

155

when you get home, then eating it within a week. It's also a good idea to shop at a deli that's busy. Faster rotation of meat and cheese through the store means it doesn't have time to sit on the shelf letting bacteria grow.

Eating raw cookie dough. Whether you mix it up at home or buy it ready to bake, raw cookie dough can be contaminated with harmful bacteria. It's meant to be baked before you eat it to kill these harmful bugs. Some of the danger comes from ingredients like raw eggs carrying *salmonella*. Protective measures like pasteurization have greatly cut the incidence of bacteria in the egg supply, but some 660,000 people still get sick from eating eggs every year.

Other risky ingredients in dough may include raw flour carrying *E. coli*. In a 2009 outbreak of food poisoning that sent 35 people to the hospital, the culprit was believed to be purchased chocolate chip cookie dough eaten raw. Although some experts recommend that raw cookie dough sold in the stores should be manufactured so it can be eaten without baking, your best bet is to keep your hands out of the bowl of dough.

Making a habit of grilling meat. That tasty charred coating on your steak or chicken is really a sign of danger. Barbecuing meat outside or even pan frying at high heat can form the cancer-causing compounds polycyclic aromatic hydrocarbons (PAHs) and heterocyclic amines (HCAs). Small changes in how you cook meat can help limit your exposure, so pick one of these methods to cut formation of PAHs and HCAs.

- Pick lean cuts of meat, which have less fat to drip onto the flames. That means fewer flare-ups and less charring.

- Marinate meats before you grill, which can cut the formation of HCAs by more than 90 percent.

- Microwave meat first, so it spends less time on the grill.

- Use a slow cooker for moist cooking of meat that concentrates the flavor without creating cancerous chemicals.

Sniffing moldy food. Mold spores can go airborne, causing breathing problems or an allergic reaction. That's why it's best to keep food with mold on it away from your face. It may be safe to cut off visible mold from certain dense foods, like hard cheese or vegetables like carrots. Then you can eat the rest. But if you see mold on more porous foods like bread or luncheon meats, toss it. Mold can spread below the surface of the food without you seeing it.

Assuming your refrigerator is the right temperature. To keep food safe, your refrigerator should stay at 40 degrees Fahrenheit or below. Cold temperatures keep bacteria in a state of suspended animation rather than allowing it to grow. But a recent survey found that more than one-quarter of U.S. household fridges were warmer than that.

To be sure, place a refrigerator thermometer in the center of a middle shelf. After about eight hours, check to be sure it reads about 38 to 40 degrees. If it's higher, lower the temperature. Of course, the temperature can vary in different parts of the refrigerator, so keep milk and eggs in the coldest part of the fridge. Don't bother using that egg rack on the door.

Rinsing off bagged lettuce. Fresh vegetables sold in plastic bags have already been washed in a chlorinated solution — sometimes more than once. If harmful bacteria have managed to survive beneath the surface of lettuce leaves after that treatment, they're not likely to be removed by a rinse in your sink.

In fact, you risk cross-contamination when you let fresh vegetables come into contact with your cutting board, sink, or colander — which may have held germier foods like raw chicken. So you can feel safe eating bagged veggies straight from the package if they're labeled "ready to eat" or "washed," but make a habit of rinsing off lettuce that's sold by the head.

Secret to food storage savings

You can save money buying ketchup or peanut butter in huge containers at the warehouse store. But can you use it up before it goes bad? Check this simple chart before you hit the grocery store so you'll know how much to buy.

Food	Shelf life after opening	Things to remember
ketchup	4-6 months in refrigerator	color or flavor may change over time, but it's still safe
jelly	1 year in refrigerator	store in fridge even before opening
mustard	6-8 months in refrigerator	color or flavor may change over time, but safe unopened for 2 years
broth	2 days in refrigerator	buy small containers, since it's good unopened for a year
peanut butter	2-3 months	lasts longest in refrigerator
mayonnaise	2 months	keep in refrigerator door to prevent separating
all-purpose flour	10-15 months	store in freezer during hot, humid weather
brown rice	6 months in refrigerator	oil in bran layer causes rancidity at room temperature
vegetable oil	3 months in pantry, 6 months in refrigerator	avoid frequent temperature changes
olive oil	12-18 months	will solidify in fridge, but it's still good
vinegar	6 months	strain out added herbs when vinegar level drops

Food	Shelf life after opening	Things to remember
soy sauce	1 year in refrigerator	evaporation will darken color and intensify flavor over time
Worcestershire sauce	2 years	color and flavor may change over time
pasta	1 year	store in airtight container in cool, dry place
coffee	1-2 weeks in pantry	freeze whole beans, but don't thaw and refreeze
sugar	indefinitely	store in airtight container in cool, dry place
brown sugar	4-6 months	will harden if allowed to dry out
honey	indefinitely	if it crystallizes, place open jar in pan of warm water
maple syrup	1 year in refrigerator	buy in glass container to prevent mold
vanilla extract	1 year in pantry	keep sealed so volatile oils don't escape
butter	3 months in refrigerator	keep in freezer if bought in bulk
canned nuts	2 weeks	unsalted and blanched varieties last longer than salted

Microwave like a pro — worry free

When it comes to cooking in the microwave, there are those who do and those who don't. In other words, some people use their microwave ovens to their full potential, cooking complete meals quickly and easily without ever turning on the stove. But others never progress beyond heating a cup of tea. Harness the full power of your microwave without worry — and without creating a huge mess in the kitchen. Steer clear of these microwave mistakes.

Making hard-boiled eggs in the microwave. It's tempting to try this trick to speed up that batch of deviled eggs. Don't do it. A whole, intact egg turns into a bomb in the microwave, sending out eggshell shrapnel and burning hot yolk and albumin when it explodes.

You can cook eggs in the microwave, but first remove them from their shells. Also break the yolks, or at least prick them with a fork. Doing this releases pressure from fluids expanding as they heat, thus preventing an explosion. For hard- or soft-boiled eggs, use the stovetop instead.

It's also best to cook eggs using medium power — say, the 50-percent power setting on your microwave. Eggs cooked on full power can get tough in one spot while another spot is still cooking.

And don't think you're safe just reheating a hard-boiled egg in the microwave. These can explode, too, even after you take them out and begin eating. A group of British eye doctors warn of the danger, recounting the story of a 9-year-old girl who suffered eye injuries when a hard-boiled egg exploded in her face. The egg had just been reheated in the microwave.

Getting careless with cheap glassware. You may be accustomed to taking your glass bakeware in and out of the oven, microwave, refrigerator, and freezer without worry. After all, brands like Pyrex and Anchor Hocking are labeled safe for these uses, right?

The truth is, glass can break when it develops tiny cracks over time, then water gets in the cracks and expands from extreme heat. So it's possible for even a Pyrex dish to shatter in the oven or crack when you remove it from the microwave.

In 2011, *Consumer Reports* reported on a 12-month study to see just how safe common glass bakeware is. It found modern Pyrex and Anchor Hocking brand bakeware tended to shatter at lower temperatures than some European brands.

Part of the problem is a change in materials. Old reliable Pyrex bakeware made by the Corning company used borosilicate to make sturdy glass, but now it's made from soda lime silicate. Some say this newer material is more likely to crack under sudden temperature changes or when a very hot or cold dish is knocked against a hard surface.

Glass bakeware made from borosilicate is still made by non-U.S. companies, including Arcuisine Elegance and Marinex. Look for these brands at online retailers like *www.amazon.com*. Or keep using your Pyrex and Anchor Hocking safely by following these precautions.

- Don't remove a hot dish from the microwave or oven and place it directly into the freezer or refrigerator.

- Don't use the browning feature when using bakeware in the microwave, and don't overheat oil or butter.

- Avoid knocking a hot casserole against a hard surface, such as your countertop, to prevent shattering. Carefully place the dish on a soft cloth or trivet instead.

- Throw out glassware that has visible cracks.

- Read and follow the directions that came with your bakeware.

Assuming vintage tableware is safe. Your old Melmac plates and bowls feel like they're made of plastic, but they may not be safe in the microwave.

Dishes made of melamine resin, like the popular Melmac tableware sold before the invention of microwaves, overheat when you nuke them. They can even singe or break in the hottest spots.

Check dishes for a "microwave safe" label or icon before you assume they can go there. If you're not sure, you can test a utensil or vessel to see if it's microwave safe.

- Fill a 1-cup glass measure with water and place in the microwave.

- Place the utensil to be tested next to — but not touching — the cup of water.

- Microwave on high power for one minute.

- If the utensil feels hot, it contains metal and is not microwave safe. Don't use it.

Risking your family's health with poisonous plastics. Bisphenol A (BPA) is used in some food containers and in the lining of food cans. It can break down when a plastic container is overheated or in certain alkaline environments, leaching out and possibly getting into food.

The U.S. Food and Drug Administration (FDA) recognizes the possible risks of BPA, but it does little to regulate its use in plastics. Based on research, those dangers might include:

- raised risk for prostate and breast cancer, since BPA functions like an estrogen in your body.

- higher risk of developing heart disease.

- greater chance of developing type 2 diabetes, likely because BPA causes endocrine dysfunction.

- liver problems, including abnormal liver enzymes and fat accumulation inside liver cells.

To stay safe, avoid using plastic containers in the microwave, but instead use glass or ceramic containers that are micro-wave safe. Look for food containers with recycle codes 2, 4, or 5, which are unlikely to contain BPA, and steer clear of those with codes 3 or 7.

And don't microwave food with plastic wrap touching it. Instead, cover your plate with an inverted plate or paper towel.

Just say 'no' to cut chemical risk

Along with cutting clutter in your purse and saving a few trees, turning down unnecessary cash register receipts may save your health.

Thermal receipts are a surprising source of the chemical bisphenol A (BPA). Researchers in Boston found some paper receipts from banks with up to 19 milligrams (mg) of BPA in a 12-inch strip.

Maybe worse, the practice of recycling paper — including receipts — means more BPA is added to recycled paper products like napkins and paper towels, spreading the danger. So if you handle a contami-nated receipt twice a day, and use other types of paper products five or 10 times a day, you would get about 2 percent of your daily BPA exposure from paper.

Don't accept a receipt unless you know you will need it. Ask if it can be emailed to you instead. If you must take one, wash your hands immediately after.

Boiling water like there's no tomorrow. "Superheating" occurs when a cup of water or other liquid gets hotter than its boiling point temperature without actually boiling. The surface of the liquid may look placid, but when you move the cup the liquid seems to explode — possibly on you. Also called "erupting," this scary event tends to happen in a squeaky-clean container.

Take these precautions to avoid being splashed with boiling liquid.

- Use a container with sloping walls, such as a glass measuring cup.

- Leave a wooden spoon or chopstick in the cup of liquid while it's heating.

- Add a pinch of instant coffee, gelatin, or a tea bag at the start or halfway through heating.

- Never cook anything in the microwave for longer than recommended.

Zapping bugs on a dry kitchen sponge. Your kitchen sponge is the dirtiest item in the dirtiest room of the house. When researchers at NSF International tested sponges from real households, they found that 77 percent were infested with coliform bacteria, a marker of fecal contamination.

In fact, sponges are so notoriously dirty that the FDA actually prohibits restaurants from using them to make a final cleaning of surfaces that come into contact with food.

You can kill germs on your kitchen sponge by putting it in the dishwasher every day, letting the high heat kill bacteria. Most sponges can also be cleaned by putting them in the microwave to kill bacteria, but you must take precautions.

Be sure the sponge is wet. A dry sponge can catch fire from overheating in the microwave. Also be sure your sponge doesn't contain any metal, like some that have a rough scrubby side. Put the wet sponge in the microwave for about a minute on full power.

Or avoid the sponge problem altogether by using a cloth dish towel and putting it through the laundry regularly.

Trying to speed up home canning. You used to be able to buy canning devices to use in the microwave, but not anymore.

Now the FDA recognizes that microwaves — and conventional ovens, for that matter — don't maintain a high enough temperature inside food to kill harmful bacteria that can grow in the canned food. A microwave tends to heat up food from the outside in, so cool spots may remain that don't get sterilized.

So when it's time to can those homegrown green beans or peaches, use a water bath or pressure canner rather than your microwave.

5 tricks to help you breathe easy

Researchers think the notoriously bad air pollution in Mexico City is damaging the brains of children and adults there, causing changes similar to those brought on by Alzheimer's disease and Parkinson's. Studies also have shown how breathing dirty air can lead to heart disease, strokes, and early death.

Tiny particles of harmful air pollutants don't just come from car exhaust or factory fumes but also from cooking, heating, and other indoor sources. Breathe easily inside your home by following these five lung-protecting rules.

Eat an apple a day. Apples and apple juice are known to reduce lung disease risk. Eating and drinking more apple products is linked with lower rates of lung cancer and other cancers. Experts say you can most likely thank the fruit's large supply of phytochemicals, including quercetin.

Research says these natural plant chemicals may also help prevent cell damage in your lungs, protect you from asthma and chronic obstructive pulmonary disease (COPD), and even help your lungs work better. One study found that female teachers in France who ate more apples had less asthma than those who ate less. Who knew the old "apple for the teacher" could do so much good?

Pick the right air purifier. Inventors have come up with several basic types of air-cleaning devices.

- UV. Ultraviolet germicidal irradiation (UVGI) cleaners use UV light from special lamps to kill live pollutants such as viruses, bacteria, and mold. They're meant to kill critters growing on the surface of HVAC ductwork, so they're not a replacement for air filters. Another type uses UV light along with a substance that reacts with a gaseous pollutant to make it harmless.

- Mechanical. These include high efficiency particulate air (HEPA) filters, designed to remove tiny particles from the air. They function as physical barriers to trap and remove pollutants.

- Ionization. These electronic air cleaners give an electrical charge to particles in the air, allowing them to be captured more easily.

- Ozone. This lung irritant is dangerous at high levels, yet ineffective as an air cleaner at low levels. The American Lung Association recommends against ozone purifiers, since they can be harmful for people with asthma.

When it comes to buying an air purifier, you don't always get more for more money. Small appliance-type air cleaners are available for around $50, but tests show they don't work that well.

On the other end of the cost spectrum are whole-house models that connect to your central air and heating unit. You'll probably pay around $1,000 to $3,000 for one of these.

A good middle ground may be one of the whole-room models that start at about $300. These can do a good job without breaking the bank. But look at the particular model's clean air delivery rate (CADR) to see if it's meant to cover the size room where you will use it. Experts say a CADR above 350 is considered excellent, while one below 100 is poor.

Cook with care. Thank goodness for modern kitchens. Cooks no longer need to breathe in smoke from a cooking fire every day while preparing meals for the family.

But cooking still has its risks. Fumes from wok cooking using oils are a major cause of lung cancer among women in Asian countries.

Cooks in the United States are also not safe. A new study investigated ways to cook on a gas stove while avoiding breathing in dangerous fumes containing nitrogen dioxide, carbon monoxide, and formaldehyde. Here's what the study found.

- Using the exhaust fan can remove up to 90 percent of air pollutants, protecting you from dangerous cooking fumes.

- But even the most popular fans aren't perfect at removing air particles. Some are so loud they inhibit conversation, although many of these models also do the best job of cleaning the air.

- Cooking on the back burners of a four-burner stove lets vents work best. Overall, the study found you can cut exposure to dangerous fumes by half by turning on the fan and using a back burner.

It's also best to avoid "ductless" range hoods, which don't vent to the outdoors. Instead, they release vapors into the house — including the same air pollutants and moisture you want to get rid of.

Keep an eye on radon. The Environmental Protection Agency (EPA) says up to 6 million U.S. homes have high levels of radon, an invisible and odorless gas that forms when uranium decays. Radon can come up from the soil and enter your home through drains, pipes, and gaps in the foundation.

Problem is, radon gas is blamed for about 12 percent of lung cancer deaths every year. It's one of the leading causes of lung cancer in nonsmokers.

To cut the danger, the EPA suggests you test for radon in all floors of your home below the third story. You can buy a testing kit for between $10 and $15 at a local hardware store. Look for a device that is state certified or contains the phrase "Meets EPA requirements." If you prefer, you can hire an accredited contractor to do the job. Find one through the website of the National Radon Safety Board, *www.nrsb.org.*

Short-term testing should be done in the lowest level of your home with the doors and windows closed. Long-term testing can take up to a year to complete, but it's the best method to determine your home's year-round average risk for radon exposure.

If you find high levels of radon, you'll need a contractor to seal cracks and holes in your home's foundation and vent radon-laden air from under the foundation.

Give dust mites the door. For people with certain health conditions, indoor pollutants like dust mites and cat dander can be a real problem. These pollutants can trigger an asthma attack or bring on an allergic reaction.

Using an air filter or air-cleaning system alone is not enough to keep the indoor air clean. Controlling the source of the problem is also important. If you're allergic to dust mites, using impermeable mattress covers works as well as using an air filter to keep air clean. If you don't have a mattress cover, try vacuuming your mattress daily and washing your sheets in hot water weekly to keep allergens under control.

Other long-term solutions include removing carpet from your bedroom and replacing it with hard flooring and keeping the relative humidity level in your home lower than 45 percent. Mites shrivel up and die in dry air. You can also treat carpets, beds, and furniture with an acaricide, a type of pesticide that kills ticks and mites.

Popular drugs may worsen asthma

About one-quarter of Americans older than 45 take statins to battle high cholesterol. But these popular drugs may actually harm your breathing if you suffer from asthma.

A recent study showed that people with asthma did 35 percent worse on breathing tests after their first year taking statins. They also used rescue medications 72 percent more than at the start of the study.

Statins change how your body makes certain immune cells, some of which increase inflammation in your airways. That's especially bad for people with asthma triggered by allergies.

Previous studies have been on both sides of the fence, with one noting statins seemed to keep people with asthma out of the emergency room. Talk to your doctor if you have asthma and are considering a statin to determine the best choice for you.

Chemical-free tips to rid your home of pests

Nearly a billion pounds of pesticides are released into the environment every year as people try to kill insects and other critters in their homes, offices, and crops. It's the never-ending struggle of man versus pests, and chemical insecticides are a powerful weapon. But these common products could be poisoning your immune system.

The idea may sound crazy, but it's not. Researchers found that women who had the most exposure to pesticides — and it's not all that much — have a greater risk for developing autoimmune diseases like rheumatoid arthritis and lupus. Some 76,000 women 50 years and older answered questions about their lifestyles and insecticide use as part of the Women's Health Initiative Observational Study.

The biggest problem seems to be with long-term exposure rather than a single episode of pesticide use. So using various types of household pesticides, living on a farm, and working with pesticides on the job nearly doubled the risk of developing an autoimmune disease for some women.

The study is not proof that these chemicals will harm you, but it's a good reason to use natural choices when possible. Here are four great options.

Mix up some vinegar magic. That old saying from Ben Franklin, "A spoonful of honey will catch more flies than a gallon of vinegar," may not actually be true. In fact, vinegar works quite well to lure flies to their deaths. Use it to keep annoying fruit flies from taking over your kitchen.

If you've ever used apple cider vinegar to wash windows, you know how flies and gnats are attracted. You can just set out a bowl of vinegar and they'll congregate. Add a teaspoon of liquid dish soap to the vinegar, and leave it out wherever you have a problem with flying insects. They'll be attracted to the vinegar and try to land, but the soap breaks the surface tension of the water so they drown instead.

You can also use vinegar to keep your pets free from annoying pests. Spray your dog daily with a half-and-half solution of vinegar and water to ward off fleas. And apple cider vinegar can work from the inside out to keep your horse comfortable. Add a few tablespoons to your horse's oats to cut down on biting flies.

Make mice skedaddle. Nobody wants to deal with dead mice caught in traps, whether they're the snapping kind or the sticky type. But you don't want to expose your family to dangerous poisons, either.

Grab that box of baking soda from the pantry and use it to deter mice. Simply sprinkle baking soda around the edges of your basement walls, in dresser drawers, or in any other places where you see evidence of a mouse. When mice return to the spot, they'll run through the baking soda. Then they'll need to clean it off their paws by licking them, so they'll swallow the baking soda. With no way of expelling the gas that builds up in the stomach, the mice will die.

Or try these other non-messy, non-bloody, non-chemical tricks to deal with that mouse in your house.

- Set out small dishes with instant mashed potato powder or buds, and put bowls of water nearby. Mice will chow down on the potatoes, then seek water to wash it down. Puffed-up potatoes in their stomach will do the trick.

- Put used kitty litter in the basement, attic, or behind the walls where you hear mice at play. Mice don't like cats — or the smells they leave behind.

- Soak cotton balls in peppermint oil and place them in mouse-prone places, such as behind electrical outlets in the wall. Mice will work hard to avoid the scent.

Put peppermint oil to the test. DIY author Terri McGraw, known to her fans as "Mrs. Fixit," points out that you get double pest-prevention power with peppermint. Along with repelling mice, this pleasant-scented oil will also stop ants cold before they can enter your home.

McGraw suggests dipping a rag in peppermint oil and stuffing it into cracks or openings to deter mice, then spraying a bit of peppermint oil around door frames. Mix up one part peppermint oil with 10 parts water in a spray bottle for a no-ant spritz.

Other strong-smelling herbs may also keep away insects. Try mint leaves, lavender, bay leaves, or citrus to keep your home smelling fresh and free of ants and other pests.

Harness power from your pantry. Insects hate the smell of cinnamaldehyde, the active ingredient in cinnamon. In fact, experts have even created a crop pesticide from cinnamon called Cinnamite. You can benefit from this remarkable natural bug repellent, too. Use cinnamon right from your kitchen cabinet to wipe out these three annoying invaders.

- Ants. These pesky critters come into the house in search of food. Find the line their columns follow, and trace it back to the point of entry. Make a barrier by sprinkling cinnamon across the path. Ants won't cross the line. You can also use chalk, ground black pepper, or turmeric as a barrier.

- Moths. It's not the ones you see gathered around a lamp that you should worry about, but the tiny moth larvae in your closets and drawers. Make sachets of cinnamon wrapped in cheesecloth to deter them from nibbling on your clothing. You can also include dried lavender or rosemary to give your closets and drawers a lovely scent. Also, be sure to clean linens and clothing before you store them. Moth larvae like fabric that's soiled with food stains.

- Silverfish. You may notice these ugly insects in the damp corners of your kitchen or scrambling around under the bathroom sink. Put a little cinnamon inside drawers and cabinets, especially in damp, warm places. Silverfish hate cinnamon and will stay away. It's also a good idea to vacuum the areas where you see silverfish to remove food crumbs and insect eggs.

Scare off mosquitoes with the power of flowers

Enjoy grilling out this summer without swarms of biting insects. And there's no need to endure toxic chemical insect repellants. A natural product derived from flowers repels mosquitoes, fleas, deer ticks, houseflies, and fire ants.

This natural plant chemical, geraniol, is made from geraniums, lemon grass, and other plants. Vegetable gardeners know to plant geraniums to ward off pests like beetles and cabbage worms.

Researchers in Florida spent 17 years testing nearly 4,000 natural chemicals to find one to rival the pesticide DEET. Geraniol was five times as effective as citronella candles at keeping away mosquitoes.

But since geraniol has also been used to attract bees for pollination, it may attract bees to you as well, so beware.

You'll find geraniol in the form of sprays, granules, infused wristbands, and towelettes from BugBand and MosquitoSafe.

Win the war against mold

The air inside your home may be 100 times more polluted than the air outdoors, according to the U.S. Environmental Protection Agency (EPA). Surprisingly, living in a new home doesn't make you safe — the air may actually be worse due to tighter seals. Mold spores thrive in a damp, enclosed space, making some parts of your home ideal for this dangerous dark intruder.

Mold spores can enter your body when you breathe in. They can also get in through your skin or when you eat food. Exposure to common household molds may lead to asthma, sneezing, runny nose, red eyes, or skin rash. One person may not be affected, while another living in the same home may have a serious reaction to common molds like penicillium, cladosporium, or strains of aspergillis mold. People with weak immune systems, including infants and elderly people along with those on certain drugs or chemotherapy, are at the greatest risk for health problems.

There's a mold fit for every surface, with varieties that grow on everything from paper and wood to carpeting and food. As long as moisture is available, mold can get a foothold. These top eight places household mold will grow may surprise you.

- closets
- flooring
- showers and tubs
- dishwashers

- windowsills
- wallpaper
- washing machines
- potted plants

Avoid the problem by following these mold-prevention tricks.

Get the wet out. It can be hard to keep moisture from building up in enclosed spaces like closets. Desiccants work by soaking up moisture from their surroundings. Some, such as silica gel or alumina, can be dried out in a 300-degree Fahrenheit oven, then used again. But other desiccants, like calcium chloride granules, can be used only once.

Another problem area for mold is underneath vinyl wall covering. Once moisture gets between the vinyl and the gypsum wallboard behind it, mold is happy to follow. You'll suspect a problem when you see pink or yellow splotches on the vinyl. Contact a professional, since this may be a sign of improper home pressurization.

In the bathroom, be sure to run the fan or open the window when you shower — and for up to 10 minutes afterward. That way the room won't stay moist constantly.

Care for your air. Mold loves to grow in temperatures of around 77 to 86 degrees Fahrenheit, so summer is its heyday. Running the air conditioner in your house works to both lower the temperature and cut the level of moisture in the air to slow mold's growth.

You can also increase the ventilation in your home by opening the windows or using a ventilating fan. But sometimes allowing air from outdoors into your house can make things worse, since it may also bring in high humidity. During the summer months, don't open your windows at night unless the temperature is at least 15 degrees cooler than the temperature your air conditioning is set at. Also be sure the dew point temperature is below 55-60 degrees. Then you won't be turning your house into a swamp.

A digital temperature and relative humidity (RH) sensor is available for about $20 at stores like Radio Shack and *www.amazon.com*. Make this small investment, and you'll know whether your indoor air is encouraging mold growth.

Don't skimp on post-disaster cleanup. After your home is flooded, mold can be a serious problem, especially on and underneath carpeting. If you can dry out wet materials within 48 hours, you may be able to prevent the growth of mold.

If the floodwater consisted of clean rainwater or water from pipes, the carpet and padding may be worth saving. But if the water included contaminated sewer water, it's probably not worth the trouble and expense of cleaning. In this case, your carpet is likely full of infectious organisms.

A good professional cleaner will remove the carpet and pad from your home, then clean and dry them at its facilities using a steam-cleaning method. But if you have small area rugs that need cleaning, just toss them in the washing machine.

Take extra care of appliances. Dishwashers, washing machines, and dryers — all appliances that get wet — can harbor mold. One study found that 35 percent of dishwashers tested were infected by a type of mold that can get into your lungs. The mold was thickest on the rubber seal around the dishwasher door.

Avoid this problem by leaving the door of your dishwasher open after you run it and wiping off moldy spots with a bleach solution. Also, be sure to run an exhaust fan or leave open the kitchen windows when you cook, run the dishwasher, or even wash dishes in the sink.

And don't neglect the laundry room. South Carolina home-owner Jennifer H. noticed a problem with mold growing inside the lid of her washing machine, which was in a storage room at the back of her home. The problem was at its worst during the humid summer months.

"We started leaving the washing machine lid open when it wasn't in use," she said. "Then the machine's metal and rubber parts could dry out, so mold didn't grow inside."

Prepare new shower curtain for a long life

Make your new shower curtain or liner last longer by keeping away those ugly mildew stains with the right preparation.

In your bathtub, mix up a batch of saltwater deep enough to submerge the curtain. Use about 2 tablespoons of salt per gallon of water in the tub, making sure the salt dissolves. Gently submerge the curtain and let it soak for 20 minutes.

Don't rinse the curtain, but hang it and let it air dry. An invisible coating of salt will penetrate the fibers, preventing mildew from growing.

Put mold killers to work. Surveys find mold growing on 80 percent of windowsills, refrigerators, shower curtains, and under sinks. There's no true "mildew killer" — a product that can kill mildew and keep it from growing back. Even worse, any chemical that claims to kill mold is also toxic to you and your pets, so use it with care.

But sometimes you have to bite the bullet and use what works. Here's how.

- Bleach. During summer, when mold is at its worst, wipe down windowsills and other key mold-growing areas once a week with diluted bleach.

- Hydrogen peroxide. You can also mix up a half-and-half solution of 3-percent hydrogen peroxide and water and put it in a spray bottle. Spritz the walls and ceiling in your bathroom, and let them dry.

- Clove oil. Mix about a half teaspoon of clove oil with a pint of water and put it in a spray bottle. You can spray and scrub it onto mold-growing zones, then let it dry to prevent more growth. Clove oil works as a mild natural antiseptic.

Don't ignore the great outdoors. Keep mold from taking over the outside of your home by preventing a buildup of water around the foundation. Inspect gutters and downspouts for leaks regularly. Make sure sprinklers are pointed away from the house — not onto the siding. Also, be sure your yard is graded properly so that water doesn't tend to run toward the foundation.

2 ways to save your cheddar

Buy a large block of cheese when it's on sale, but take care to keep it fresh until you can use it all. Here are two ideas for preventing mold and extending the life of your cheese.

Smear on some butter. Apply a light coating of butter to the cut edges of a block of cheese before you put it in a plastic bag. This seals out the air, so mold spores won't grow.

Salt it down. Take a paper towel or napkin, soak it in saltwater, then wrap it around a block of cheese to protect the cut edges from air. Again, no more mold.

Take precautions in the greenhouse. Molds like botrytis can grow on your plants and in their soil. It can enter the wounds of plants to stunt their growth. Keep these greenhouse blights in check by cleaning up dead leaves and plant matter, allowing for good air circulation around plants, and removing standing water that can increase the humidity near plants. Your geraniums will thank you.

DIY laundry formulas give stains the heave-ho

Some popular brands of laundry detergent are so expensive, they're used as currency on the "black market." Police report that people are stealing multiple bottles of the detergent to resell it. If you're in charge of doing the laundry for a good-sized family, you know the pain of paying $20 for a big bottle of name-brand detergent.

But you don't have to pay through the nose to have clean clothes. When you buy commercial cleaning products, you're paying for the brand name and fancy packaging. Make your own all-purpose cleaners and stain removers with these simple formulas. These four homemade mixtures work just as well as the brand-name products at a fraction of the cost.

Vinegar mixture gets out tough stains. You can buy a 16-ounce bottle of white vinegar for less than $2 — a lot less than you'd spend on that much detergent. Even better, you avoid exposing your family to harsh, unhealthy chemicals when you use this natural wonder. Vinegar works in the wash to soften your clothes and break down detergent residue. Simply add a cup to the final rinse.

You can also use vinegar as a stain remover. Mix together vinegar, water, and a bit of liquid detergent in a spray bottle and use it to pretreat stains like perspiration, ring-around-the-collar, and even stains from deodorant.

Treat a wine stain quickly with vinegar, and you may be able to remove it from cotton or cotton-blend fabrics to save that special blouse. Sponge full-strength white vinegar directly onto the stain, then rub away the wine spot. Launder as usual.

Vinegar is also your best bet when it comes to keeping colors from running in new clothes. Soak those new blue jeans or brightly colored towels in vinegar for about 15 minutes before washing them for the first time. Your jeans will stay dark, and towels won't fade.

Beware these sudsy substitutions

If you've ever made the mistake of using liquid dish soap — the kind for washing dishes in the sink — in the dishwasher, you know that not all soap substitutions work out well. Make this mistake, and you're likely to spend time cleaning up suds from the kitchen floor.

The same thing goes for laundry substitutions. In a pinch, you may be able to hand wash a blouse using shampoo or liquid dish soap. Their degreasing power may remove a greasy food stain.

But don't think you can use any old household soap or detergent in the washing machine. The wrong products can lead to oversudsing and a soapy mess. You may also have trouble getting residue out of your clothes.

Never put these cleansers in your washing machine.

- dishwasher detergent
- dishwashing soap
- shampoo
- bubble bath
- ammonia

Lemon juice makes great rust remover. Blend together lemon juice and salt. Rub the paste onto a spot of rust on your favorite shirt, and watch the spot disappear.

Remember putting lemon juice on your hair in the summer to help it lighten in the sun? The same principle works in the laundry room. You can whiten whites that can't be bleached by adding one-quarter cup of lemon juice to the washing machine. Of course, don't use lemon juice on silks.

Baking soda deodorizes — just like in the fridge. Move this 99-cent item from the kitchen cupboard to the laundry room, and let it save you money while getting your clothes clean and fresh.

First, sprinkle a little baking soda into the bottom of the laundry hamper or even right onto dirty clothes, and you can avoid that funky smell until washday comes.

Then, you can deodorize your clothes and linens by adding one-half cup of baking soda to the rinse cycle of the washing machine.

A half cup of baking soda along with your regular detergent can also remove dirt and grease from clothes and get them cleaner and brighter. Minerals in the baking soda help neutralize the wash water to help detergent do its job. You may even be able to cut in half the amount of bleach you use.

And some people save money by using baking soda to mix up their own version of a popular laundry booster and stain treatment. One frugal Indiana homemaker finds this blend works like a dream to clean her husband's greasy clothes, soiled from metalworking in the garage.

Mix together a quarter cup washing soda, a quarter cup baking soda, and a half cup hydrogen peroxide. Use this handy blend as a pretreatment for stains, or add each ingredient separately into the washing machine.

Cornstarch is a stain lifesaver. That other box of white powder in your pantry also does great things in the laundry room.

You can use cornstarch to get out stains, including those ugly rings on shirt collars and an errant spot of blood. Mix a paste of cornstarch and water, then apply it to the stain, let dry, and brush off the excess.

Also, since the laundry starch you buy is made mostly of cornstarch, it's no surprise that you can mix up your own version. In a spray bottle, blend a tablespoon of cornstarch into two cups of cold water. Shake well before using.

Use TLC with your HE washer

New high-efficiency (HE) washing machines use less water to wash clothes, saving you money on water and energy. But follow instructions about what products to use.

Your washer's manual probably says to use only detergents and fabric softeners labeled for use in an HE machine. Using non-HE products — like the regular detergent you have left from your old machine — can cause excess sudsing, buildup of mildew in the machine, and clothes that don't get clean.

But you can use some of the same traditional laundry boosters in an HE machine as long as you add them correctly.

- Vinegar. Put in fabric softener dispenser so it's added during the rinse cycle.

- Baking soda. Sprinkle into washer over clothes before you start the load.

- Borax. Sprinkle into washer, making sure to break up any clumps.

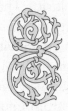

Anti-aging tricks to look great and feel even better

Beauty trends with ugly consequences

You look good now, but you may feel much worse later. Making a fashion statement sometimes means making a questionable choice about your health. Watch out for these treacherous beauty trends that put style over safety.

Sidestep high heel problems. High heels may lead to high medical bills. That's because these stylish shoes can be a real pain. Here are some of the issues associated with high heels.

- Arthritis. Iowa State researchers found that regularly wearing and walking in high heels can contribute to joint degeneration and knee osteoarthritis. It also alters your posture and puts a strain on your lower back. The higher the heel, the greater the risk.

- Muscle strains. Women who wear high heels often experience discomfort and muscle fatigue. A Finnish study suggests that long-term high heel use may also increase the risk of injuries. That's because wearing high heels changes the way you walk — even when you're no longer wearing them. Habitual high heel wearers put much greater stress on their calf muscles rather than on their more elastic tendons when walking. This can boost your risk of muscle strain injuries.

- Hammertoe. Stuffing your feet into high heels can also lead to hammertoe, a painful condition in which your toes bend in on each other. While you can buy pads and gel protectors to treat hammertoe, you may need surgery to correct it.

- Ingrown toenails. High heels represent one of the most common causes of ingrown toenails. With your toes crammed into high heels, your big toenail may grow into the skin. An ingrown toenail not only hurts, it can also become infected and may require the removal of the entire nail.

To protect yourself from these painful problems, consider giving up high heels entirely. If that's not possible — or desirable — take some precautions to lessen your risk of complications.

- Wear comfortable shoes on your commute to work, then change into high heels when you arrive. At the end of the day, ditch the heels and put the comfortable shoes back on. Use the same strategy for parties, weddings, and other formal events.

- Shop wisely. When shopping for shoes, avoid overly pointy, tight footwear. Look for those with plenty of room for the toes and good arch support. Try shoes on for 10 to 15 minutes to make sure they're comfortable.

- Put new shoes to the cutout test. Trace your foot on a piece of cardboard, and bring this cutout with you when shopping for shoes. If you can't fit the cutout into a shoe without bending or crumpling it, then your foot will end up suffering.

Get the lead out. Pucker up for lead poisoning. That could be what you're doing when you put on lipstick. A recent U.S. Food and Drug Administration (FDA) study found that over 400 popular lipstick brands contain more than twice as much lead as expected.

Because lead builds up in your body over time, applying lipstick every day — or several times a day — could add up to dangerous levels. As a known brain toxin, lead can cause learning, language, and behavioral problems.

In the wake of this study, the FDA may set a maximum limit of allowable lead in lipstick. But in the meantime, consider using less of it. And keep your lipstick out of the reach of young children so they don't play with it.

Blunt nail salon risks. You may pamper yourself with a trip to the nail salon for a manicure or pedicure now and then. But while you're making your nails pretty, you may also be exposing yourself to surprising dangers.

- Polish perils. Your nail polish may contain dangerous chemicals. A recent report by California's Department of Toxic Substances Control found harmful toxins even in nail products labeled "nontoxic."

  Researchers tested 25 products for the so-called "toxic trio" of dibutyl phthalate (DBT), toluene, and formaldehyde. Exposure to these chemicals has been linked to cancer, birth defects, asthma, and other health problems. Alarmingly, some of the nail products that claimed to be free of DBT or toluene had even higher levels of these chemicals than the products that made no such claims.

While workers in poorly ventilated salons are most at risk, salon customers and consumers should also take note. You may consider using less nail polish or going to the salon less often to limit your exposure.

- Skin cancer scares. If your salon uses an ultraviolet (UV) nail lamp to dry your nails, you may be at greater risk for skin cancer. Recently, two case studies suggest that these UV light boxes may be linked to skin cancer of the hands.

  While the evidence is scant, it's still troubling. Salons often use UV lamps to dry gel manicures, acrylic nails, and even regular nail polish. You may be better off sticking to a traditional polish, or lacquer, and letting it air dry.

Shrug off purse pain. Oversized purses may be stylish, but they can cause back pain, shoulder stiffness, headaches, poor posture, and stiff necks. This happens because the purse's weight pulls down on your shoulder, straining your neck and the nerves that exit the neck and line your shoulder.

To ease this strain, clean out your purse every week. Reorganize the remaining contents so all the pockets get used. This helps distribute weight more evenly. Clean out your wallet, too. Carry only the cash and credit cards you need. Also, don't always carry your bag on the same shoulder. Alternate between shoulders or cradle the purse in front of you in both arms.

Minimize makeup mishaps. A seemingly good trend can have unintended bad results. That's the case with makeup that contains sunscreen. While it's good to know your foundation or tinted moisturizer provides some protection from the sun, it would be a mistake to rely on these cosmetics alone. They simply don't provide enough protection — and a false sense of security could lead to skin cancer.

Instead of counting on your makeup to protect you, make sure to put on sunscreen, too. You should apply it to your face, neck, ears, hands, and any other exposed skin.

Pay attention to more than just the SPF number. Also look for the term "broad spectrum" on sunscreen products. This indicates that the product blocks both ultraviolet A (UVA) and ultraviolet B (UVB) rays. UVB rays cause sunburn, while UVA rays penetrate deeper and trigger premature aging. Both contribute to skin cancer.

Edible beauty products promise tasty results

Not all beauty trends are dangerous. The latest trend involves nutricosmetics, beauty products that you eat or drink rather than apply to your skin.

Nutricosmetics are currently much more popular in China and Japan, where you can munch on collagen-infused marshmallows, but they are gaining steam in the United States.

Available products include Beauty Booster, an antioxidant-rich elixir that you drizzle over foods or into drinks, and Nimble, a nutrition bar that nourishes your skin. You can sip a variety of beautifying beverages, including four kinds of Skin Balance waters, and even snack on Skin Balance Gummi Bears.

Like other beauty products, these edible beauty boosters come with steep price tags. And they may not be necessary. Most doctors do not recommend them, noting that you can get the same skin-enhancing benefits from fruits, vegetables, and water.

Foods that make you look younger

You can spend big bucks on beauty products to try to look younger. Or you can simply tweak your diet to achieve the same results for a fraction of the cost. Discover the "beauty foods" — they naturally keep your skin young, your bones strong, your hair healthy, and your smile sunny.

Nix these skin-aging no-no's

Refuse to look old before your time by refusing to indulge in foods that can speed up the aging process. Limit or avoid the following items:

- fried foods

- sugar

- salt

- alcohol

- soft drinks

- processed and refined foods

- junk food, such as candy and potato chips

Go green with tea. Sip a soothing cup of green tea to stave off wrinkles. You'll see why drinking this is like sipping from the mythical "fountain of youth." It actually prevents your cells from aging.

Research shows that the polyphenols in green tea protect your skin from the harmful effects of ultraviolet radiation. These include skin cancer, sunburn, and photoaging — the damage done to your skin from prolonged exposure to the sun and other sources of UV light. Signs of photoaging include wrinkles, dark spots, and leathery skin.

Unlike sunscreen, green tea does not block UV rays. Rather, it works at the cellular level to reduce sunburn cells and fight off inflammation that contributes to the aging of your skin.

One recent study found that drinking a beverage rich in green tea polyphenols for three months helped women's skin, improving skin hydration, density, smoothness, and elasticity. It also boosted blood flow to the skin, which may contribute to its positive effects.

You don't even have to drink tea to reap its benefits. Other studies show that applying it topically also provides protection from UV rays and fights signs of aging. But, of course, that's not as satisfying as drinking it.

Cook more tomatoes. Forget injections and creams — there's an inexpensive veggie that boosts your skin's collagen naturally. And it can cut your chance of heart disease by a third, too. It's the tomato, and it gets its power from the mighty antioxidant lycopene.

In a small British study, 20 women received either 55 grams of tomato paste mixed with olive oil or olive oil alone each day for 12 weeks. Researchers found that tomato paste protects against the damaging effects of ultraviolet radiation in the short term and possibly for longer. Among the benefits was an increase in procollagen, the precursor of skin-strengthening collagen. Women in the tomato paste group got 16 milligrams of lycopene daily.

That's not just good news for their skin, but also for their hearts. A large study of more than 39,000 middle-aged and older women found that higher blood concentrations of lycopene meant a lower risk of heart disease. Women with higher-than-average lycopene levels reduced their risk by 34 percent compared to women with the lowest levels.

Tomatoes contain more than just lycopene. They also provide other carotenoids, vitamin C, potassium, and fiber in a low-calorie package. Raw tomatoes make a tasty snack or a fine addition to salads or sandwiches, but tomato sauce and tomato paste give you more lycopene. That's because heat and oil allow your body to absorb more of it.

If you prefer to drink your tomatoes, opt for organic tomato juice when possible. A Spanish study found that organic tomato juice contains more polyphenols than juice from conventionally grown crops.

Pump up with iron-rich foods. Thinning hair could mean you need more of one nutrient — iron. Research suggests a possible link between hair loss and iron deficiency, especially in women. Low levels of iron in the blood may make hair loss worse or speed up the process. Fortunately, boosting those iron levels may help re-grow hair or at least stop the shedding.

While iron supplements are available, they should not be taken without a doctor's supervision because too much iron can lead to a dangerous condition called iron overload. The best way to get it is through eating more of these iron-rich foods — lentils, beans, oysters, clams, spinach, prunes, raisins, tofu, and lean beef.

If you're a woman suffering from thinning hair, ask your doctor about a blood test to check your iron and red blood cell levels.

Don't forget your morning OJ. Need more calcium? Here's the convenient and refreshing way to get it every day without dairy products or calcium tablets. Just drink a glass of orange juice. One cup of calcium-fortified orange juice gives you 50 percent of your daily calcium needs. Calcium helps keep your bones strong, reducing your risk of osteoporosis, breaks, and fractures and improving your posture.

And pay attention to wrinkles. Women with wrinklier skin may be more likely to have brittle bones. In a recent study of 114 women in their late 40s and early 50s, those with the worst wrinkles on their faces and necks also had the weakest bones.

Vanquish varicose veins with vitamin K

Worried that your legs may look like road maps? Follow this simple route to prevent varicose veins. Eat more dark leafy greens, which are loaded with vitamin K.

French researchers found that a protein dependent on vitamin K may play a role in the development of varicose veins, a condition marked by an achy and unsightly tangle of swollen blue veins.

The matrix Gla protein (MGP) normally blocks the calcification, or hardening, of veins — but this lab study found that, in varicose veins, calcification and an incomplete, inactive form of MGP were both present. Because MGP requires vitamin K to become activated, researchers suspect that low vitamin K levels could be to blame.

Boosting your intake of foods rich in vitamin K may get MGP working properly again, allowing you to ward off varicose veins. Good sources of vitamin K include spinach, kale, collard greens, turnip greens, and broccoli.

Fortify with fruit and fish. Here's a winning combination to keep you grinning with confidence. Fiber from fruit and omega-3 fatty acids from fish may help you maintain healthy gums.

In a recent study of 625 healthy veterans with an average follow-up of 15 years, men aged 65 and older who ate more high-fiber fruits were less likely to show signs of gum disease. For each serving of high-fiber fruit, the risk of tooth loss dropped by 12 percent, the risk of receding gums dipped by 5 percent, and the risk of bone loss in the part of the jawbone that supports your teeth fell by 14 percent.

The extra chewing required to eat high-fiber foods could boost saliva production, which helps remove harmful bacteria from the mouth. Fiber may also help by controlling blood sugar and lowering blood pressure, since poorly controlled blood sugar and high blood pressure are risk factors for gum disease.

However fiber helps, it can't hurt to eat more fruit. Good high-fiber choices include bananas, apples, oranges, blueberries, raspberries, blackberries, pears, strawberries, prunes, and dates.

Several studies suggest that omega-3 fatty acids fight gum disease, thanks to their anti-inflammatory powers. One recent review of eight previous studies determined that long-chain omega-3 fatty acids — the kind found in fish oil — show promise as a treatment for gum disease. A study of more than 9,000 people found a link between higher dietary intakes of omega-3 fatty acid, especially docosahexaenoic acid (DHA), and a lower risk of gum disease. And a Japanese study found that a higher intake of DHA may slow the progression of gum disease in older people.

To get enough omega-3, aim for two fatty fish meals per week. Salmon, mackerel, herring, or tuna should do the trick.

Wash it down with water. Drink plenty of water to defeat dry, damaged skin. When you drink water, you moisturize your skin from the inside out, making it soft, supple, and pliable rather than parched and droopy. One way to see if you're drinking enough is to pinch the skin on the back of your hand. If it doesn't spring back into place, you need to start drinking more.

It's a good idea to carry water around with you. But bottled water is not necessarily any better than tap. Unlike cities that supply public water, bottled water makers don't have to tell you what contaminants they find during testing, how or if water has been purified before bottling, or where the water originally comes from. See the feature *Better alternative to bottled water* for more information.

Foods that fight wrinkles

Eating foods rich in these nutrients can help defend against aging.

- A high concentration of carotenoids in your skin may mean fewer furrows and wrinkles, a German study found. These brightly colored antioxidants fight damaging free radicals produced by ultraviolet radiation. You'll find them in cantaloupe, apricots, carrots, sweet potatoes, and spinach.

- Ellagic acid may stop skin wrinkling and the inflammation that leads to photoaging. That's what Korean researchers discovered in a series of lab tests using human skin cells and mice. Eat more berries and drink pomegranate juice to reap these benefits.

- Choose foods rich in vitamins A, C, and E and the minerals zinc and selenium. They may ward off wrinkles by zapping free radicals. That means eating plenty of colorful fruits and veggies like squash, papayas, mangoes, peaches, oranges, kiwifruit, red bell peppers, and broccoli. Enjoy low-fat milk, eggs, nuts, seeds, and fortified whole-grain cereals as well.

Better alternative to bottled water

It's a shocking secret of the nation's beverage industry — half of all bottled water is just fancy, dressed-up tap water. Manufacturers may run tap water through a filter before bottling, to remove the taste of chlorine, but don't expect it to be healthier or even safer than what comes out of your own faucet.

In 2008, the nonprofit Environmental Working Group (EWG) tested 10 brands of bottled water and found that some of these popular drinks were contaminated with urban wastewater pollutants, drugs like Tylenol, minerals such as arsenic, radioactive compounds, fertilizer residues, industrial chemicals, and byproducts from chlorine, some of which have been linked to cancer. One brand of bottled water even promoted the growth of breast cancer cells in a lab study.

The Food and Drug Administration regulates bottled water safety, but in some ways the standards are less strict than for tap water. Your best bet for safety and savings is to drink filtered tap water. Tap water suppliers must publish the results of their water quality tests. Call your local water agency and find out which contaminants, if any, were found in your water. Then buy a faucet-mount or pitcher-style filter made to capture them. Visit the website *http://www.ewg.org/tap-water/getawaterfilter* for help in choosing a filter.

If you can't give up bottled water, protect your health by choosing a brand whose label:

- shows it is certified by the National Sanitation Foundation (NSF).

- tells you the water's geographic location and source.

- says it has been treated with an advanced purification method, such as reverse osmosis, to remove contaminants.

- lists a contact phone number or website where you can get the results of water quality tests.

Look lovely for less

You use your kitchen to cook delicious meals or bake tasty treats. But your kitchen can also help you whip up amazing homemade beauty products. Save hundreds of dollars a year with these easy, cost-effective tips.

Help your hair. Beautiful hair can be yours, thanks to everyday items from your kitchen. Check out these nine nifty natural ways to gorgeous hair.

- Rosemary. Rosemary can make your hair appear shinier. Steep two rosemary tea bags in a cup of hot water for 10 minutes, then pour it into a spray bottle. Spritz the rosemary tea onto your hair after you wash it. Your hair will reflect more light and look dazzling. As a bonus, rosemary also helps soothe your dry, itchy scalp. The oils in rosemary may boost circulation, which relieves dryness.

- Vinegar. Give your hair shine and bounce with a vinegar rinse. Mix half a cup of apple cider vinegar with two cups of warm water, and pour over your freshly washed hair. The vinegar rinse gets rid of the gunk that builds up from hair spray, gel, and other styling products.

- Thyme. When it's time to fight dandruff, turn to this fragrant herb. Boil two tablespoons of dried thyme in a cup of water for five minutes. Let the mixture cool, strain it, and massage the liquid into your hair and scalp to stop the flaking. Don't rinse. Just let this simple remedy do its job.

- Tomato juice. Keep your hair looking and smelling great with tomato juice. To remove odors, such as smoke, massage a cup of tomato juice into your hair and rinse twice — once with warm water and again with cool water. Soaking your hair in tomato juice also helps remove chlorine and gets rid of the greenish tint that blondes may acquire from the pool. Rinse out the juice in the shower after about 10 minutes.

- Baking soda. Remove all the residue from hair spray and styling gels with baking soda. Just blend about a tablespoon of baking soda with your regular shampoo. Or mix a tablespoon of baking soda with a cup of water and massage it into your hair and scalp. It will strip away the film in your hair, leaving it shiny and bouncy. Just be careful not to get any baking soda in your eyes.

- Flat beer. It may not be tasty to drink, but flat beer can give your limp hair a lift. Flat beer strips away soapy film and brings new life and bounce to your hair. Mix three tablespoons of flat beer in half a cup of warm water, and pour it over your head during your shower. It will give your hair extra body. Cheers!

- Honey. Give your hair a thorough conditioning. Massage a quarter cup of honey into your scalp, and cover your hair with a plastic bag for at least 15 minutes. Then rinse with hot water.

- Bananas. Fix your dry hair by mashing a banana with a tablespoon of almond oil and rubbing the mixture into your hair. Leave it there for 20 minutes, then rinse.

- Avocados. Follow this recipe for shiny hair. Mash an avocado with a tablespoon of olive oil and a teaspoon of baking powder. Massage the mixture into your hair, and let it sit for 15 minutes. Then wash your hair and watch it shine.

Save your skin. Forget costly creams, facial masks, and oint-ments. Make skin care products right in your own kitchen. Don't skip this chance to save money while improving your skin.

- Oatmeal facial. This amazing natural treatment smoothes and refines your skin and pores — plus it can even out your skin tone for a youthful look. Research has shown that beta-glucan from oats can penetrate skin and fight wrinkles. Oatmeal also removes surface impurities, restores your skin's moisture balance, acts as a gentle facial scrub, and soothes sensitive or irritated skin.

   Here's how you can take advantage of oatmeal's soothing, smoothing powers. Just add a handful of dry instant oatmeal to your regular facial cleanser, and pack it on your skin. Gently scrub it off after 10 minutes.

   For oily skin, make a mask using dry oatmeal and an egg white. Mix until it feels sticky, then apply it evenly to your face and leave it on for 15 minutes. For dry skin, mix a cup of oatmeal with a mashed ripe banana, and add enough milk to make a paste. Apply it to your face, and leave it there for 10 to 15 minutes. As a bonus, it will also exfoliate your skin.

- Mayonnaise mask. If you have dry skin, try this simple trick. Use whole-egg mayonnaise, and apply it to your face. Leave it on for 20 minutes, wipe off the excess, and rinse with cool water.

- Yogurt night cream. Wake up to smoother skin when you use this homemade night cream. Simply squeeze half a lemon into a cup of plain yogurt and stir. Then raid the refrigerator each night for a dollop of this mixture. Rub it onto your face before bed, just like you would your

197

regular night cream. After three to four weeks, you'll notice healthier-looking skin.

Bask in the powers of olive oil

Looking for an all-purpose beauty aid in your kitchen? Reach for the olive oil. This healthy oil works wonders for your hair, skin, and nails.

- Pour half a cup each of olive oil and boiling water into a large glass jar with a lid, and shake well. Let cool slightly and massage it into your hair. Cover your hair with a shower cap or plastic bag, and wrap your head in a hot towel. After half an hour, shampoo as usual.

- For stronger nails, soak them in warm olive oil for 10 minutes. Your nails will be less prone to chip and peel.

- Mix equal parts salt and olive oil, and gently massage your face and throat for five minutes. Then wash your face. Your skin will have a radiant, golden glow.

Be nice to your nails. Pamper your nails in the comfort of your own home with these simple tricks.

Make your own cuticle cream by mixing two teaspoons of petroleum jelly, half a teaspoon of olive oil, and a quarter-teaspoon of lemon juice. Dab a little on each nail and rub it into your cuticles each night before bed.

To make your manicure last longer, clean your nails with cotton balls soaked in vinegar before you polish them.

5 habits for a healthy mouth

Keep your dazzling smile well into your golden years by taking care of your teeth and gums. Brushing, flossing, and making regular trips to the dentist serve as the building blocks of good oral hygiene. But you can go beyond the basics with these helpful tips.

Be gentle. The most common mistake people make when brushing their teeth is brushing too hard. You may even have been taught to do this — but it can ruin your gums. Instead of vigorously scrubbing your teeth, brush very gently for two to three minutes. Concentrate on brushing just two teeth at a time rather than swiping long strokes across several teeth.

Choosing the right toothbrush can help. The American Dental Association (ADA) recommends using a toothbrush with soft bristles. That's because hard, stiff bristles can wear away your enamel — your teeth's hard outer coating — and damage your teeth and gums.

An electric toothbrush can also do the trick. Plus it also comes in handy if you have limited ability to move your shoulders, arms, and hands. Studies have found that an oscillating rotating power toothbrush works better than a manual one when it comes to removing plaque and reducing gingivitis. Because the brush heads rotate in one direction and then the other, this type of brush does a good job of reaching all the nooks and crannies in your mouth.

Rub it in. Sometimes, you don't need a toothbrush at all. Your finger will do in a pinch. A recent Swedish study found that using toothpaste as a lotion and massaging it onto your teeth — in addition to your usual morning and evening brushings — works just as well as brushing three times a day.

This technique could be a simple, low-cost way to give your teeth an extra dose of fluoride during the day. Keep this tip in mind for after lunch, when you may not have a toothbrush handy.

Just remember that the "massage" method is an extra step. You should still brush your teeth every morning after breakfast and every evening before bed.

Minimize mouth odors. Give bad breath the boot with the potent mouthwash you can make from your pantry. Just add a half-teaspoon of baking soda and a half-teaspoon of salt to a cup of water. Then rinse it around your mouth for an effective — and cheap — weapon against bad breath.

Baking soda neutralizes odors caused by bacteria rather than masking them. In fact, a University of Nebraska College of Dentistry study found that baking soda worked just as well as hydrogen peroxide or a combination of hydrogen peroxide and baking soda to prevent the growth of oral bacteria in lab tests. Salt, or sodium, also acts as a disinfectant to kill germs.

Unique way to whiten your teeth

Characters in silent movies or cartoons might slip on a banana peel and fall. It's a reliable old gag that can still make you smile. But here's a new, unusual use for banana peels that will also leave you smiling.

Instead of monkeying around with expensive whitening strips, use a banana peel to whiten your teeth. Simply peel a ripe banana, and rub the inner white side of the peel against your teeth for about two minutes each day. You can do it before or after you brush your teeth.

How does it work? Your teeth may absorb the minerals in the peel, including potassium, magnesium, and manganese. Or it could be the acids in the peel, which lighten stains without damaging the enamel.

However it works, it just might be worth a try. You may end up with a brighter smile after about a week.

Pop some peppers. Toothpaste and mouthwash aren't the only things you should put in your mouth to keep it healthy. Make room for an occasional sweet green bell pepper, the vegetable with 35 percent more vitamin C than an orange. It also has tons of vitamin K, vitamin B6, and more. Eating these babies will battle arthritis, squash your lung cancer risk, and save your teeth.

Bell peppers also come in red, orange, yellow, and even purple. These bright colors don't just make your dishes more vibrant. They also deliver two nutrients that protect your teeth. A small Japanese study discovered that people who get more of a particular group of nutrients may be less likely to lose their teeth. Vitamin B6 was one of these crucial nutrients, and bell peppers help you get more. Peppers also provide plenty of vitamin C, and many gum specialists recommend vitamin C for healthy gums. Vitamin C's ability to repair the connective tissue in gums may help protect your teeth, too.

But the benefits of bell peppers extend far beyond your mouth. As a rich source of vitamin K, green peppers may help you avoid disabling osteoporosis and osteoarthritis. Research suggests that people whose diets contain lots of vitamin C and beta cryptoxanthin, a phytochemical found in abundance in red peppers, have lower risks of developing inflammatory polyarthritis — inflammation of more than one joint — and lung cancer.

Snack on fresh, raw peppers, or add them to salads. Fill a whole, lightly steamed pepper with rice pilaf, or add chopped peppers to stir fries, stews, or Cajun foods. You can even roast red peppers to add tangy flavor to pasta. However you choose to eat peppers, it's a good idea to add more of these colorful and healthy veggies to your diet.

Avoid acidic foods. On the other hand, you may want to limit acidic foods and drinks that can damage your enamel. Culprits include soft drinks, sports drinks, energy drinks, sour candy, and vinegar. Citrus fruits, berries, and many fruit juices are also acidic, but because of their nutritional benefits, you shouldn't avoid them entirely. Just be aware of their acidity.

After consuming acidic foods or beverages, wait at least 30 minutes before brushing your teeth. You'll give your softened enamel time to harden again, which lessens the chance of damage. Another trick is to drink milk or eat cheese rich in calcium before or during meals to help strengthen your enamel.

Check your mirror for warning signs

Unlike the wicked queen in "Snow White," you probably don't have a magic mirror on your wall. But your ordinary mirror can still provide plenty of important information. Simply gazing into your looking glass may help you face facts about your health. Next time you're primping, pay attention to these red flags.

Open your eyes to possible danger. Your eyes may be the window to your soul — but they also give you a glimpse at your overall health. Here are four signs that your eyes could be warning you of a serious illness.

- Raised yellow patches on your eyelids. You'd be surprised what your eyes can tell you about your heart. Look for this telltale sign that indicates you're on a fast track to high blood pressure, heart disease, or stroke.

  Called xanthelasmata, these yellow cholesterol deposits are not painful or harmful. But they are unsightly. And, according to a recent Danish study, they could boost your risk of heart disease or heart attack. Among men ages 70 to 79, those with xanthelasmata had a 12 percent higher risk of heart disease compared to men without the condition. The risk was 8 percent greater for women in the same age group.

- Droopy eyelid. If your eyelids seem to droop, it may simply be a sign of aging. But if you have trouble closing one eye or controlling your tears, it could be Bell's palsy, a temporary paralysis in half your face caused by an impairment of the nerve that controls facial muscles. Half of your face may appear droopy, and the affected eye may either produce excessive tears or no tears at all.

  In rare cases, droopy eyelids may also be a sign of an autoimmune disease called myasthenia gravis, which weakens muscles throughout the body, or even a brain tumor.

- Bulging eyes. Yikes! Your reflection looks like you've just seen a ghost. Or you're doing your best Don Knotts impression. Bulging eyes are most likely caused by hyperthyroidism, or an overactive thyroid. The most common form is Graves' disease. Too much thyroid hormone causes the tissue around your eyes to swell, making you look bug-eyed. Other symptoms include weight loss, nervousness, and sweating.

- Yellow eyes. When the whites of your eyes look more like yolks, it's called jaundice. And it can be a sign of liver disease. The yellowing occurs because of a buildup of bilirubin, a byproduct of the breakdown of red blood cells. A healthy liver whisks away waste products like bilirubin, but conditions like hepatitis or cirrhosis impair your liver's ability to work properly.

See a doctor if you notice any of these eye-related symptoms. Diagnosis and treatment can have you looking — and feeling — out of sight.

Heed your hair. Your hair, believe it or not, holds secrets about you. These shocks from your locks can tell you about nutritional deficiencies or medical conditions. You won't even need a fine-toothed comb to search for the following clues.

- Dandruff. Brush away these flakes by brushing up on your diet. Dandruff may be the result of a nutritional deficiency. If you have dry skin along with your dandruff, aim for more essential fatty acids, such as omega-3 from fatty fish, flaxseed, and nuts. Boosting your intake of B vitamins and zinc should also help.

- Dull, limp hair. Trying too hard to lose weight? You may lose some luster from your hair, too. Very-low-calorie diets may not provide enough nutrients, leaving your hair dull and limp. They can even stunt hair growth. Make sure you're eating enough protein, iron, omega-3 fatty acids, zinc, and vitamin A.

- Hair loss at an early age. If your hair is a distant memory, remember to watch out for prostate cancer. A recent French study suggests that men who started going bald at age 20 are more likely to develop prostate cancer later in life. In the study, men with prostate cancer were twice as likely as men without the disease to have started losing their hair when they were 20. But if you started going bald in your 30s or 40s, there was no added risk. Because early balding may be a risk factor for prostate cancer, consider getting screened for the disease if you started losing your hair at a young age.

- Prematurely gray hair. Going gray before age 40 is usually no big deal — especially since you can mask the gray by coloring your hair. But in some cases, gray hair could be caused by anemia, thyroid problems, or a vitamin B12 deficiency. If prematurely gray hair does not run in your family, consider looking into these possibilities.

- Thinning, brittle hair. Hypothyroidism, or an underactive thyroid, could be to blame. When your thyroid gland doesn't produce enough thyroid hormone, your hair could pay the price. Other symptoms of hypothyroidism include being more sensitive to cold, constipation, depression, fatigue, joint or muscle pain, paleness, dry skin, weakness, and unintentional weight gain. A mineral deficiency could also be the culprit. Make sure your diet includes enough magnesium, selenium, and silica.

Nail down nail problems

You don't need a mirror to examine your fingernails, but you should still polish up on these warning signs.

- Brittle nails. Nails that dry out and crack could be a sign of hypothyroidism. They could also indicate a diet low in iron.

- Pitted nails. Small dents or pits in your nails could mean psoriasis, a skin condition characterized by scaly red patches.

- Yellow nails. If the whole nail looks yellow, it could be a sign of lung disease or diabetes. Yellow spots could signal fungus or psoriasis. Red nail beds are another symptom of diabetes.

- Peeling nails. Nails that peel easily could mean your diet lacks linoleic acid. You can find it in vegetable oils.

Foolproof remedies for puffy eyes

Your eyes look like they're going on a long trip — because they have plenty of baggage. Puffiness, bags, and dark circles under your eyes make you look old and tired. Luckily, you can take a vacation from puffy eyes with remedies found right in your own home. Find out how to make the puffiness disappear in the blink of an eye.

Spoon out some relief. A cold spoon can serve your swollen eyes well. Stick a spoon in a glass of ice water for about 30 seconds. Then hold the curved back of the spoon against your eyes. You can also keep a handful of spoons in the refrigerator for this purpose. That way, you can replace each spoon with a fresh cold one as it starts to warm up.

Push back with produce. One garden variety remedy is to place cold, crisp cucumber slices on your eyes for about 15 minutes. The coolness and moisture will help reduce swelling — and you'll feel like you're at a spa getting pampered.

Potatoes can also provide a solution. To combat dark circles under your eyes, cut a raw potato into half-inch slices, and place them over your eyes for about 20 minutes. Enzymes in the potato help lighten discolored skin, while the coldness constricts blood vessels to reduce pooling, which can make the circles even darker. You can also peel and grate a potato, then wrap it in a towel to make a poultice to lay over your eyelids. The starch from the potato has anti-inflammatory effects to soothe sore eyes.

Even frozen veggies work. You can use a package of frozen peas or corn as an eye mask. Just wrap the bag in a soft, dry cloth, then lay it over your eyes.

Crack the case with eggs. Beat puffy eyes by beating an egg white in a bowl. For an extra boost, you can add a drop or two of witch hazel. Using your fingers or a soft brush or cloth, dab the foamy egg white mixture under your eyes, and let it sit for about 15 minutes before rinsing. The egg white will make your skin feel tighter and look less puffy, while the anti-inflammatory witch hazel will also squelch puffiness.

Try a little tea. When you wake up with puffy bags under your eyes, it's tea time. Brew yourself a pot of chamomile tea. Chamomile is a naturally soothing herb that temporarily decreases puffiness. Just ice the tea, soak a washcloth or a couple of gauze pads, and place them over your eyes.

Don't worry if you don't have chamomile. Any tea should do the trick. Herbal teas, including chamomile, soothe redness and inflammation. But caffeinated teas also help by constricting blood vessels and reducing swelling.

Deflate those puffy eye bags with tea bags. Steep two tea bags in hot water for a few minutes, and let them cool. Then place the tea bags over your closed eyes.

Turn on the tap. Make a splash in your battle against puffy eyes. Soak your face in a bowl of ice cold water. The cold water causes your blood vessels to constrict and the swelling to go down. Pressed for time? Simply splash some cold water on your face. This trick works well in a pinch.

Stir in some salt. Eating too many salty foods can leave you with puffiness around your eyes — but salt can also be the solution to the problem. Just stir a teaspoon of salt into two cups of hot water. Dip some cotton balls, pads, or a clean cloth into the solution, and place them over the puffy areas. The warm salt water will wash away the swelling.

Opt for oil. Try this bright idea to lighten those dark circles under your eyes. Dab a bit of castor oil under each eye twice a day. The unsaturated fatty acids in castor oil help lock in moisture and plump up the thin skin. That way, the underlying bluish blood vessels won't show through as much.

Prevent bags with simple changes

You'll find lots of ideas on how to treat the bags under your eyes. But the best way is to sidestep the problem before it strikes.

- Get your allergies or hay fever treated. They could be the source of all your troubles.

- Drink plenty of water. Drinking water helps ward off dehydration. When you're dehydrated, you retain fluids and look puffier.

- Limit alcohol, which dehydrates you and weakens the skin around your eyes.

- Steer clear of salty foods. A high-sodium diet can cause water retention and puffiness.

- Get enough sleep. Maybe your eyes look tired because you're worn out.

- Sleep on your back with an extra pillow. This keeps excess fluid from pooling under your eyes.

- Give your eyes a rest when using the computer or watching TV for long periods of time. Aim for a five-to-10-minute break every hour.

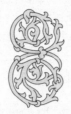

Can't miss body-slimming solutions

Trick your tummy to feel full, longer

Curb overeating and cure those snack cravings. The right foods and habits can satisfy your appetite, quiet hunger, and fill you up so you eat less.

Enjoy eggs for breakfast. Eat protein in the morning, and you'll eat less all day. A healthy breakfast, especially one rich in protein, makes you feel fuller and reduces hunger throughout the day.

Brain scans in one study showed that a high-protein breakfast quieted the brain signals that motivate you to eat all the way until lunch time. "Incorporating a healthy breakfast containing protein-rich foods can be a simple strategy for people to stay satisfied longer, and therefore, be less prone to snacking," says Heather Leidy, assistant professor in the University of Missouri's Department of Nutrition and Exercise Physiology.

But don't limit this strategy to breakfast. Eating a little lean protein at each meal can help fight hunger when you're trying to lose weight. Men who did that felt fuller throughout the day and had less desire for a late-night snack. They also had fewer thoughts about food.

"Our advice for people trying to lose weight is to add a moderate amount of protein at three regular meals a day to help appetite control and the feeling of fullness," says Wayne Campbell, a professor of foods and nutrition at Purdue University.

Stick to lean sources of protein — for instance eggs, beans, and lean pork, like Canadian bacon. Fatty meats can fill you up, too, but they'll sabotage your weight loss.

Turn to green tea. A cup of green tea with dinner could make you less likely to go back for seconds. In a small study, people who drank a cup of hot green tea after a turkey sandwich still felt fuller two hours later than those who drank hot water. Taste is key. Green tea has flavor; water does not. Scientists think flavor increases your perception of being full and keeps you feeling satisfied.

That's not all this ancient drink does. It's chock-full of antioxidants that may play a role in preventing cancer and heart disease. Plus, it could slash your risk of diabetes and boost your cells' sensitivity to insulin.

Supplements may not be the same boon to weight loss. In fact, they could threaten your health because they:

- generally contain lots of caffeine.

- may harm your liver.

- interfere with some medications, including MAO inhibitors for depression and proteasome inhibitors for multiple myeloma.

Some of them are poor quality, too. Two out of six green tea supplements failed testing by an independent laboratory. Neither contained the amount of active ingredients their labels claimed. One contained much more caffeine than it claimed, the equivalent of two cans of cola. The other contained dangerous amounts of lead.

Don't waste your money on these supplements for now. Stick with the real thing, and enjoy watching the weight slide off.

Pop the perfect snack. The next time you want to indulge in a snack, reach for popcorn. A 100-calorie serving will fill you up better than 100 calories of milk chocolate, according to research.

It can even be healthy. "Popcorn may be the perfect snack food," notes Joe Vinson, professor of chemistry at the University of Scranton. "It's the only snack that is 100 percent unprocessed whole grain. All other grains are processed and diluted with other ingredients." Ounce for ounce, popcorn also boasts more polyphenol antioxidants than fruits or vegetables.

Just watch what kind you buy and how you cook it. Popping it in oil, pouring on the butter, or making a batch of sweet kettle corn can kill its health benefits. "Air-popped popcorn has the lowest number of calories," Vinson explains. "Microwave popcorn has twice as many calories as air-popped." So does popping the kernels in a pan of oil.

Cut into kumquats. Naringenin, a simple compound in citrus fruits like grapefruits and kumquats, may be the next big thing in weight loss.

In mice fed a fatty, American-style diet, adding naringenin to their food:

- reprogrammed their liver to burn excess fat instead of storing it.

- lowered cholesterol.

- normalized blood sugar metabolism.

- stopped weight gain, even on a high-fat diet.

Normally, these mice would become seriously overweight. Not this time. "The marked obesity that develops in these mice was completely prevented by naringenin," says Murray Huff, the study's leader and Director of the Vascular Biology Research Group at the University of Western Ontario. He notes that the effects did not come from calorie intake since all the mice ate the same amount. And the animals didn't curb their appetites or eat less food, which are often the ways people try to prevent weight gain and the metabolic conditions that result.

Kumquats are a can't-beat source of naringenin, as are grapefruits, grapefruit juice, tangelos, and pummelos. You can't get the amount of naringenin in this study purely from food, but eating fruits naturally rich in it won't hurt. Eat kumquats whole — peel, seeds, and all. The skin is sweet while the pulp is tart, making for a tasty combination.

Sip before meals. The grapefruit diet used to be all the rage, but now science says water is just as effective at helping you shed pounds. Plus, it's free and right at your fingertips.

People were assigned to eat half a grapefruit, drink 4.5 ounces of grapefruit juice, or drink 4.5 ounces of water 20 minutes before each meal. All of them, even the water drinkers, naturally ate 250 to 500 fewer calories every day. Yet no one felt hungry. As a result, they lost more than 7 percent of their total body weight in just three months.

Researchers were shocked. They thought people would drop more pounds on the grapefruit diet, thanks to the fruit's naturally filling fiber. Turns out, the amount of water in the fruit — or beverage — matters more. That means snacking on anything high in water and low in calories before a meal could help you lose weight.

Healthy food could sabotage your diet

Too much of a good thing can still be bad. Turns out, you can eat too much fruit while dieting. After all, it still contains calories.

"I have had many patients tell me that they don't know why they are not losing weight. Then they report that they eat fruit all day long. They are almost always shocked when I advise them to watch the quantity of food they eat, even if it is healthy," says Brooke Schantz, a registered dietitian with Loyola University Health System.

On the other hand, nonstarchy vegetables are pretty hard to overeat, since they're mostly fiber and water. Just don't load them with cheesy, buttery sauces, Schantz says. Do limit starchy veggies like peas, corn, and potatoes.

Focus on Zzz's. Not sleeping enough can actually make you hungrier. Sleep deprivation upsets your balance of leptin and ghrelin, the brain chemicals that control your appetite. These recent studies show what can happen when you don't get enough zzz's.

- Cutting their sleep back to four hours for two nights made people 23 percent hungrier during the day. They especially craved high-carb foods.

- People who got two-thirds of their normal amount of sleep ate an extra 549 calories a day. You'd gain an extra pound in one week, at that rate.

- Those who got too little sleep for two weeks in a row ate more snacks, particularly at night.

Make every effort to get enough good-quality sleep. Find clever tips to help drift off in the chapter *Best ways to beat fatigue and boost energy.*

Feel indulgent. If you think you're eating an indulgent food, you'll feel fuller. A new milkshake study proves your mind can fool your stomach.

Researchers gave people a milkshake, then they lied about it. They told some people they were getting an "indulgent," high-fat shake with 680 calories. They told others the opposite, that they were getting a "sensible" shake with only 140 calories. In reality, they all contained 380 calories.

After the shakes, researchers measured people's levels of ghrelin, a hunger hormone. Everyone should have had the same levels since they ate the same number of calories. Not so. Surprisingly, people who thought they ate the rich, fatty shake experienced a bigger drop in ghrelin, meaning their stomachs felt fuller.

"This study shows that mindset can affect feelings of physical satiety," says Alia Crum, of Yale University's department of psychology. "The brain was tricked into either feeling full or feeling unsatisfied. That feeling depended on what people believed they were consuming, rather than what they actually were consuming."

The secrets to long-term success

The strategies that help you lose weight in the beginning won't help you keep it off long-term, according to new research. For that, you need different tactics.

Five hundred women were divided into two groups, each following a different weight-loss plan. Researchers checked on their progress after six months and again four years later. Then they figured out which habits were most successful.

- Big changes like eating more fish and less fried food and dining out less boosted weight loss in the short-term.

- Smaller changes like adding more fruits and vegetables and eating less meat and cheese had a bigger impact in the long run, however.

"People are so motivated when they start a weight-loss program. You can say, 'I'm never going to eat another piece of pie,' and you see the pounds coming off," says Bethany Barone Gibbs, of the University of Pittsburgh's Department of Health and Physical Activity.

"Eating fruits and vegetables may not make as big a difference in your caloric intake. But that small change can build up and give you better long-term results, because it's not as hard to do as giving up french fries forever."

Short-term success can motivate you, but keeping the weight off can be the hardest part. So focus on habits guaranteed to succeed long-term, rather than on habits that will give you quick results.

"The focus must be on long-term strategies. Changes in eating behaviors only associated with short-term weight loss are likely to be ineffective and unsustainable."

Melt away belly fat faster

Where you tend to put on weight may matter more than how much you weigh. "When it comes to increased health risks, where fat is deposited is more important than how much fat you have," according to Cris Slentz, an exercise physiologist at Duke University.

Belly fat is by far the worst kind. It's been linked to high triglycerides and blood pressure, low levels of "good" HDL cholesterol, and glucose intolerance — all symptoms of a dangerous condition called metabolic syndrome. Belly fat also:

- makes your body resistant to the effects of insulin, which controls your blood sugar levels.

- cranks up inflammation throughout your body, a culprit behind heart disease.

- makes you more likely to die from diabetes, high blood pressure, or heart disease.

- makes you more likely to die, period.

Fortunately, you aren't at the mercy of the spare tire around your middle. These foods can naturally help you lose weight and tighten your belt to the next hole.

Snack on cereal. Melt away belly fat in just five minutes each evening. Not by doing sit-ups, but by replacing your normal evening snack with a bowl of cereal.

Thirty-five overweight people did this for six weeks. Every two weeks they were weighed and had their waists measured. Turns out, they actually ate fewer calories in the evening when they switched to cereal as a nighttime snack. They also shed pounds and shrank their waistlines, compared to the 35 people who kept eating their normal evening snack.

Choose a cereal high in fiber and nutrients but low in added sugar. The fiber in cereal may guard your body against heart disease, metabolic syndrome, and inflammation. Whole-grain cereals like bran are best. Top it off with skim or low-fat milk.

Drizzle on safflower oil. This amazing oil causes belly fat to virtually slide right off your middle. Great news if you have a lot to lose. It's a top source of healthy fats called polyun-saturated fatty acids, or PUFAs. In fact, safflower oil packs the most PUFAs and the least saturated fat of any other oil. Getting as little as one-and-two-thirds teaspoons a day helped obese women with diabetes:

- shed up to 4 pounds of fat around their middle.

- add as much as 3 pounds of muscle.

And all in just four months. These women didn't change anything else about their eating habits, nor did they start exercising. That means it might work for anyone.

"I never would have imagined such a finding," says Martha Belury, the study's senior author and professor of human nutrition at Ohio State University. "The women in the study didn't replace what was in their diet with safflower oil. They added it to what they were already doing. And that says to me that certain people need a little more of this type of good fat — particularly when they're obese women who already have diabetes."

Safflower oil also improved the women's blood sugar, as measured by their HbA1c levels; reduced inflammation; and boosted their HDL cholesterol by 14 percent.

Belury suggests using it in an oil-and-vinegar salad dressing or in cooking. It's a perfect base for a dressing because it doesn't become solid when chilled. Plus it has a high smoking point, so you can use it to fry or sauté. Don't try to reuse it, though. It goes rancid quickly after heating.

Switch to enriched orange juice. Drop pounds around your waist simply by sipping three 8-ounce glasses of fortified OJ every day.

Heavy people tried this trick for four months, drinking Minute Maid orange juice fortified with calcium and vitamin D. Each 8-ounce glass boasted 350 milligrams (mg) of calcium and 100 International Units (IU) of D. Amazingly, they lost three times more belly fat than those on regular juice.

Being low in vitamin D may encourage your body to form fat. In fact, there's a definite link between low blood levels of D and too much body fat. Calcium, on the other hand, may squash hunger and help your body flush fat out of its system.

Find the fat-burning spice. Add a dash of red pepper to your food to help your body melt away fat. People who don't normally eat spicy foods seem to get a calorie-burning boost from red pepper. They automatically ate 66 fewer calories at their next meal after eating tomato soup laced with half a teaspoon of the spice.

"We found that consuming red pepper can help manage appetite and burn more calories after a meal, especially for individuals who do not consume the spice regularly," says Richard Mattes, professor of foods and nutrition at Purdue University.

The spice especially quelled their hunger for fatty, salty, and sweet foods. It boosted metabolism, too, a lift that helped them burn an extra 10 calories. That burn in your mouth is responsible for hunger control and the spike in metabolism, says Mattes. "The burn contributes to a rise in body temperature, energy expenditure, and appetite control," he explains.

It's not a long-term weight-loss solution, since the effect seems to wear off as you get used to eating spicy foods. Once it becomes familiar to people, it loses its benefit. Still, it's an easy, delicious way to give your diet a jump-start.

Better way to predict your weight loss

There's nothing more frustrating than setting a weight-loss goal, eating right and exercising, and still not meeting it. Now a new calculator can help you set more realistic deadlines for losing weight.

Unlike old calculators, this one takes into account the fact that your metabolism slows down as you shed pounds, and that exercise makes you gain muscle, offsetting some of the weight you lose in the form of fat. Check it out online at *www.pbrc.edu/research-and-faculty/calculators/ weight-loss-predictor*.

- Type in your age, height, gender, and current weight.

- Select how many calories you plan to trim each day through diet and exercise.

The graph will show you how long it will take at that rate to meet your goals. Play with the calorie slider to see how eating more or fewer calories will affect the speed of your weight loss.

Foolproof fixes to stop overeating

Low-fat, low-carb, high-protein — even the best diet can fail if you eat too much of the foods it allows. So how do you satisfy your stomach and still shed pounds? By eating smart and tricking your belly into feeling full.

Don't be fooled by food labels. Before you crack open that can of soup or pint of ice cream, check the serving size. It's the first thing you should look for on any nutrition label. It's even more important than the fat, sodium, or calorie content.

Manufacturers sometimes suggest ridiculously tiny portions, far less than you probably eat in one sitting. This makes their product look healthier than it really is. The Center for Science in the Public Interest (CSPI) recently did some sleuthing. The worst offenders? Canned soup, ice cream, coffee creamer, and aerosol nonstick cooking sprays.

Take Campbell's condensed Chicken Noodle Soup. Sixty percent of people eat the whole can in one sitting. But the label says there are 2.5 servings per can. Shrinking the portion size allows Campbell's to claim their soup contains only 890 milligrams (mg) of sodium per serving. Eat the whole can, however, and you get a whopping 2,390 mg, more than you should get in an entire day.

Tricks like this can lead you to underestimate how many calories you're truly getting each day, not to mention how much sodium, saturated fat, and trans fat. Don't fall for it. Check the suggested serving size on labels and the number of servings in each package.

Practice portion control. Packaged foods are only part of the problem. It's all too easy to misjudge how much dinner you're dishing up onto your plate.

Experts talk about the importance of portion control, but their advice doesn't help unless you know what a normal portion looks like. Keep this list as a handy guide for common foods.

Amount of food	Size equivalent
1 ounce of chips or pretzels	one large handful
1/2 cup of ice cream	tennis ball
1 bagel	hockey puck
2 tablespoons of peanut butter	golf ball
1 small baked potato	60-watt light bulb or computer mouse
1/2 cup of cooked pasta or rice	a cupped palm
1 cup of pasta	tennis ball
1/4 cup of dried fruit or nuts	large egg or golf ball
1 medium piece of fruit	baseball
1/2 cup of cooked or raw vegetables	one rounded handful
1/2 cup of beans	bulb portion of a light bulb
1 ounce of cheese	two dominoes or a thumb
3 ounces of meat, poultry, or fish	woman's palm or deck of cards
1 tablespoon of salad dressing	half a walnut shell

Plan your plate color. Making spaghetti with tomato sauce tonight? Serve it up on a white plate. Alfredo pasta? Red or blue plate. When your meal is the same color as the plate it's on, you tend to eat more. Pick contrasting colors for your food and dishes, and you may automatically eat less.

In one new study, people were allowed to serve themselves as much food as they wanted. When they spooned food onto a plate with a contrasting color, they served themselves 21 percent less food than when they used plates that matched their meals. Eating off of a different colored dish makes portions look larger.

Even your tablecloth can have an impact. Servings shrunk 10 percent when people ate on a tablecloth that contrasted with their plate color.

TV *can trip up weight loss*

Seeing junk foods ads during your favorite shows could have you reaching for a bag of chips without realizing it.

Seventy-five people watched a 30-minute film loaded with ads for either junk food, health food, or nonfood items. Afterward, everyone rated their desire to eat. Some craved food more strongly after the junk-food laden film. Ads for health food had no effect on appetite.

The next time a commercial for fast food or fatty snacks comes on during your favorite show, change the channel. Or record your shows and fast-forward through the commercials.

Avoid distractions. Eating while doing something distracting, like watching television, leads people to eat more food than they would otherwise. Now research shows it can cause you to overeat at later meals, too.

People who played solitaire on the computer while eating lunch ate nearly twice as much food during snack time a mere 30 minutes later, compared to people who ate their lunch with no distractions. They also had a tougher time remembering what they ate, and they felt less full afterward. Experts suspect two things are at work.

- Activities distract you from the sensations of eating and feeling full. As a result, you tend to overeat.

- Distractions also affect your memory of what and how much you ate. Usually the memory of food from one meal triggers you to eat less at the next one.

This could help explain why watching lots of TV has been linked to obesity, and why obesity is such a fast-growing problem in the United States. A separate study found that overweight women ate half of all their meals in a room with the TV on.

Fight back. Don't eat meals or even snacks in front of a television, computer, or while doing other activities like reading or listening to music. Minimize your distractions. Focus on what you're eating, and you may eat less.

Slice food into smaller pieces. You'll trick your brain and your belly into thinking you've eaten more than you really have. It's a clever way to avoid overeating high-calorie or otherwise unhealthy foods.

Researchers gave 301 people bagels. Some were whole, others cut into four pieces. After eating their bagel, they were given a complimentary lunch. Those who got the whole bagels ate more food, and therefore more calories, at lunchtime than people who ate their bagel in pieces.

Your brain thinks that more pieces equal more food, so you generally feel fuller after eating something cut, sliced, or diced. Devina Wadhera, the study's lead author, suggests using this trick when you want to spoil yourself with a high-calorie food.

"Cutting up energy-dense foods into smaller pieces may be beneficial to dieters who wish to make their meal more satiating while also maintaining portion control," she says. You'll be able to eat less of it and still enjoy.

Satisfy your sweet tooth without gaining a pound

Yes, you can have your cake and eat it, too. There's no need to swear off sweets. Just follow these secrets to a happy diet, backed by science.

Eat sweets for breakfast. Believe it or not, eating dessert as part of a balanced breakfast could actually help you lose weight and keep it off long-term. Breakfast may be the best time to treat yourself for three reasons.

- Your metabolism is highest in the morning.

- It gives you the rest of the day to work off the extra calories.

- Eating breakfast does more to suppress ghrelin, a hormone that boosts hunger, than any other meal of the day.

In a new study, obese people who added cookies, cake, or chocolate to their breakfasts for eight months lost an average of 40 pounds more than dieters who avoided those types of treats. Plus, they kept the weight off longer.

Both groups ate the same number of calories each day — 1,600 calories for men, and 1,400 for women. But the sweets-eaters got more of their calories at their morning meal. They ate a 600-calorie breakfast with plenty of protein and carbohydrates, compared to the other group's low-carb, 300-calorie breakfast.

After four months, people in both groups had lost an average of 33 pounds. In the study's second half, however, those eating the low-carb breakfast regained 22 pounds, while the big-breakfast eaters lost another 15.

Experts say allowing yourself to eat a dessert early could help control your cravings all day. "The participants in the low-carbohydrate diet group had less satisfaction and felt that they were not full," explains Daniela Jakubowicz, professor of medicine at Tel Aviv University. As a result, their cravings for sugar and carbs became intense, and they eventually cheated on their diet. "But the group that consumed a bigger breakfast, including dessert, experienced few if any cravings for these foods later in the day."

Be sure to include good-for-you foods as part of your morning meal. Cake alone won't fill you up until lunch time. Successful dieters in this study ate dessert along with protein-rich foods like eggs or low-fat milk.

Sniff some chocolate. Getting a whiff of dark chocolate can quell your hunger for it. Researchers asked six women to smell dark chocolate, and six other women to eat it. Sniffing it suppressed their appetites just as well as eating it did, but without the calories. The women who merely smelled the chocolate experienced a drop in their levels of ghrelin, which made their hunger disappear. Try it yourself the next time you get hungry. Bear in mind, this study used very dark chocolate with 85 percent cocoa. Other types, like milk chocolate, may not have the same effect.

Eat dessert more often, not less. Turns out, it's better to indulge in dessert throughout the week when you're dieting than to splurge only once a week. At least, as long as your treat is sugar-free and low in fat.

The best desserts have a low glycemic index (GI) and a low glycemic load (GL). That means they raise your blood sugar slowly rather than in a rush. Obese and overweight kids who ate a low-GI, low-GL dessert every day lost more weight over three months than kids who ate the dessert of their choice only once a week. They also saw bigger improvements in their systolic blood pressure and insulin resistance — when your cells don't respond normally to insulin and glucose.

Use the tips on cutting fat in comfort foods and cooking with sugar substitutes elsewhere in this chapter to whip up a menu of waist-whittling goodies.

Sweeten with real sugar. Getting small amounts of table sugar throughout the day could help you manage your weight. Danish researchers studied more than 3,000 men between the ages of 53 and 75. Those who used real sugar in their tea and coffee were least likely to be obese.

Table sugar is made of sucrose, a combination of fructose and glucose molecules. Studies suggest eating even small amounts of glucose may:

- make you feel fuller.
- cause you to eat fewer calories.
- help control your appetite.

This study doesn't prove that sugar can help you shed pounds, but it does suggest that putting a little sugar in your tea or coffee is safe, even when you're trying to get trim.

The same is not true of sodas, unfortunately. People in the Danish study drank around six cups of coffee or tea each day, with two lumps of sugar each. That's a total of 125 calories from sugar, less than in one can of sugary soda. So ditch the soda and stick with hot tea, instead.

Take a short walk. A 15-minute walk could cut the amount of chocolate you eat in half. Workers who took a brief walk ate half as much chocolate as normal, even when they were under stress. They went from eating an ounce of chocolate to snacking on half an ounce, about the size of a "fun size" chocolate bar.

"We know that snacking on high-calorie foods, like chocolate, at work can become a mindless habit and can lead to weight gain over time," says Adrian Taylor, professor of sport and health sciences at the University of Exeter in Great Britain. Going for a walk helps break the habit.

"People often find it difficult to cut down on their daily treats, but this study shows that by taking a short walk, they are able to regulate their intake by half."

Sugar-free treats can still harm teeth

Sugar alcohols like xylitol in sugar-free sweets can help prevent cavities. But they're often paired with acidic ingredients that can eat away the enamel protecting your teeth.

The problem lies with fruit-flavored candies, gum, and soft drinks. The flavoring itself is acidic. The longer it stays in contact with your teeth, the worse the erosion. Lollipops and slow-dissolving candies are some of the biggest culprits.

Check the ingredients in sugar-free treats and diet drinks. Avoid those that list ascorbic, adipic, glutaric, or tartaric acid. Flavors such as peppermint, spearmint, butterscotch, and mint-chocolate chip are not acidic and are most likely safe.

Comfort foods that won't kill your diet

Eating low carb? Be careful. Carbohydrates help keep you happy. The right ones can even help you live longer and lose weight. Switch to whole-grain pasta, and you can enjoy your carbs and still stay trim.

Carbohydrates boost your brain's level of serotonin, a mood-regulating chemical. Low serotonin levels are linked to depression and anxiety, and it turns out a low-carb diet may affect your mood. One study found that, after a year, people on a low-fat diet that allowed carbs were happier than those on a carb-cutting plan, even though both groups lost the same amount of weight.

So instead of eliminating all carbohydrates, make a push to eat healthier ones. Whole grains are a great place to start. Out of more than 72,000 women, those who ate a diet focused on whole grains, vegetables, fruits, legumes, fish, and poultry were least likely to die from any illness, especially heart disease. Plus, the type of fiber found in whole grains seems to help prevent weight gain, particularly in the form of belly fat.

Buy the whole-grain versions of spaghetti, lasagna noodles, and elbow macaroni, for instance. Make a few more simple switches like this, and you can eat your favorite comfort foods and still watch your waistline.

Spaghetti. Begin with whole-grain pasta, then opt for a delicious, chunky, vegetable-based sauce instead of the normal meat sauce. Cut up chunks of zucchini, onion, mushrooms, and green bell pepper to beef it up without meat.

Healthier homemade ice cream

It's a summertime tradition you shouldn't have to miss. This low-calorie version makes sure you won't. Make your ice cream with low-fat milk instead of whole milk. Thicken it with unflavored gelatin to get the same texture, and get ready to enjoy a creamy, dreamy treat.

Mac and cheese. Use whole-grain elbow pasta, then whip up one of these light cheese sauces.

- Top the pasta with feta cheese and olive oil instead of cheddar and butter for a Greek twist.

- Steam then puree half a head of cauliflower. Mix with one cup of skim milk, a pound of low-fat shredded cheese, and a quarter-cup of Parmesan. Stir together with cooked pasta, pour into a casserole dish, and top with a sprinkling of bread crumbs. Bake at 350 degrees 15 to 20 minutes for a crisp, golden crust.

Cream sauces. Don't give up on pasta alfredo. Whisk one cup of low-fat milk with four teaspoons of all-purpose flour in a saucepan over medium heat. Use in place of heavy cream in your favorite cream sauces.

Casseroles. Lower the calories in each serving simply by adding more vegetables. Choose bulky ones rich in fiber and water, like celery, carrots, and eggplant.

Don't use cream soups like cream of mushroom as a filler. Make your own, instead. Mix together two-thirds cup of light sour cream, one-quarter cup of light mayonnaise, two teaspoons of mustard, and pepper and herbs to taste.

Meatloaf and hamburger. Choosing lean ground beef or turkey is a good start, but you can do much more to lighten up these staples.

- Beef up your meatloaf by mixing cooked brown rice and diced bell peppers and mushrooms into the ground meat. Use up to one cup of grains or veggies per pound of ground meat.

- Moisten meat by adding egg whites instead of whole eggs.

- Add bulk to burgers with whole bread or oats instead of bread crumbs. Run oats through a food processor before adding to meat.

- Opt for ground bison instead of beef, if you can afford it. Bison (buffalo) typically contains less saturated fat, which makes for healthier burgers.

- Top your burger with fat-free sliced cheese. Soak the cheese for two minutes in water to hydrate it, and it will melt perfectly.

Potato salad. Don't give up on your favorite summer food just because of its fat. Just use low-fat, Greek-style yogurt, which is thicker than regular yogurt, in place of mayonnaise.

Fried chicken. Even if you fry it in a healthy oil like canola, fried chicken ends up full of fat. Cut the calories by crisping it in the oven.

Dip chicken in low-fat buttermilk, low-fat milk, or egg. Then coat it in flour seasoned with pepper and spices. Bread crumbs will do the trick, too. Place on a wire rack or baking sheet, and spray the chicken with a canola-based cooking spray. Bake at 425 to 450 degrees for 30 minutes or until crispy and cooked through.

French fries. Stir up a healthy, homemade version with white or sweet potatoes. Slice into fry-size pieces, and toss in a bowl with a tablespoon of olive or canola oil. Add a dash of salt and pepper, then bake at 450 degrees for 20 to 30 minutes. You can add rosemary to white potatoes or cinnamon to sweet potatoes for extra oomph.

Brownies. Cut the fat and sugar while keeping the rich flavor. Blend a can of black beans until liquid. Use in place of oil, eggs, and other ingredients in brownie recipes. Add a little water to the batter, if needed, to reach the right consistency.

Chocolatey treats. Replace chocolate with baking cocoa to trim the fat. Use three tablespoons of cocoa in place of one square (1 ounce) of unsweetened chocolate, or in place of half a cup of semisweet chocolate. The mixture will be dry, so add:

- a tablespoon of water or applesauce when substituting for unsweetened chocolate.

- two tablespoons of water plus three tablespoons of sugar for semisweet chocolate.

Baked goodies. Reduce the butter, margarine, shortening, and oil in recipes. Swap out solid fats with half that amount of fruit puree, such as canned pears, peaches, apricots, or plums. For oils, use three-quarters the amount called for. Add more puree if the batter seems dry.

Lower-fat versions may bake faster. Try dropping the temperature by 25 degrees, and check on them a few minutes early.

Breads. Pack more nutrients into muffins, bread, and sturdy cookies by exchanging half the all-purpose flour with whole-wheat flour. For delicate cookies, light cakes, and pie crusts, opt for whole-wheat pastry flour.

Hidden facts about sugar substitutes

Confusion and controversy swirl around sugar substitutes. Are they safe? Can they help you lose weight? The answers may surprise you.

Non-nutritive sweeteners (NNS) — aspartame, saccharin, sucralose, stevia, acesulfame-K — are much, much sweeter than sugar, so you need less of them to get the same sweetness. Because they're needed in such small amounts, they add few or no calories to foods and beverages.

Sugar substitutes may not aid weight loss. Since they contain fewer calories, you'd think they would help you lose weight. In theory, they can. "While they are not magic bullets, smart use of non-nutritive sweeteners could help you reduce added sugars in your diet, lowering the number of calories you eat," says Christopher Gardner, associate professor of medicine at Stanford University. "Reducing calories could help you attain and maintain a healthy body weight ... But there are caveats."

Sure, they lower calories, but if you compensate by eating more food elsewhere in your diet, you've canceled out those savings. "For example, if you choose a beverage sweetened with non-nutritive sweeteners instead of a 150-calorie soft drink, but then reward yourself with a 300-calorie slice of cake or cookies later in the day, non-nutritive sweeteners are not going to help you control your weight because you added more calories to your day than you subtracted," he explains.

You may not consciously realize you're eating more food, though. Some research suggests that foods sweetened with NNS don't make you feel full the same way sugar-sweetened foods do. You could end up overeating because you still feel hungry.

Beverages like diet sodas sweetened with NNS don't seem to cause this problem, so switching to diet drinks may be more effective for cutting calories than eating diet foods. A few other concerns continue to dog artificial sweeteners.

- They are so sweet that they may desensitize your body and brain to the natural sweetness of foods.

- Eating foods made with them may confuse your brain into thinking that all sweet foods are low in calories, which could lead to weight gain.

Substitutes are key for controlling diabetes. Despite their spotty record with weight loss, NNS can help you manage your blood sugar. This makes them an important tool for people with diabetes. "For example, soft drinks sweetened with non-nutritive sweeteners do not increase blood glucose levels, and thus can provide a sweet option for those with diabetes," says Diane Reader, a registered dietitian and expert with the American Diabetes Association. Keep in mind, though, that foods sweetened with zero-calorie NNS may be high-fat or unhealthy in other ways.

Surprising sources of saccharin

Many over-the-counter medicines, both solid pills and liquids, use saccharin as a sweetener but don't list it on the label. One chewable aspirin or acetaminophen, for instance, may contain as much saccharin as a can of diet soda.

Pay attention if you develop itching, eczema, a rash, or if your skin suddenly becomes more sensitive to sunlight. You may be suffering an allergic reaction to hidden saccharin.

Sugar-free foods can still raise blood sugar. Don't confuse sugar alcohols with non-nutritive sweeteners. Sugar alcohols (sorbitol, mannitol, xylitol, isomalt, and hydrogenated starch hydrolysates) do contain calories and carbohydrates, although fewer than sugar. That means they will raise your blood sugar. Carefully check the ingredient list on packaged food.

While you're at it, look at the "Total Carbohydrate" content on the Nutrition Facts panel. Even if a food is made with a carb-free NNS, it can still contain sugar-boosting carbohydrates from other sources.

Some substitutes have side effects. No, aspartame does not lead to memory loss. And saccharin doesn't cause cancer. But experts have documented allergies and side effects related to a few sweeteners.

- Sugar alcohols can cause stomach problems, including diarrhea, if you eat too much of them.

- Aspartame may trigger headaches and migraines in some people, especially if used for a long period of time.

- Saccharin is made from sulfonamide, the same compound as sulfa drugs. So if you're allergic to sulfa drugs, you may have a reaction to saccharin.

Besides specific sweeteners, some studies link beverages made with non-nutritive sweeteners, like diet sodas, to a higher risk of coronary heart disease. Other research disagrees. Drinking two or more diet sodas a day may also increase your risk of kidney disease.

You can cook, even bake, with NNS. Sugar does more than sweeten foods. It also affects their volume, texture, moisture, and ability to brown. Don't cut all the sugar in a given recipe to begin with.

Start by substituting half the sugar with a non-nutritive sweetener in baked goods. Check this chart for additional tips.

Sucralose (SPLENDA)	Substitute one cup of granulated sucralose per cup of sugar.
	Consider using a sucralose-sugar blend sold in stores, instead of straight sucralose, for baked goods.
	Baked goods bake faster with sucralose. Check cakes seven to 10 minutes early, and cookies, brownies, and quick breads three to five minutes early.
	For recipes that call for lots of sugar, like frostings, candy, and fudge, replace only one-fourth of the sugar with sucralose.
	To help cakes and baked breads rise, add half a cup of nonfat dry milk powder and half a teaspoon of baking soda for every cup of sucralose.
	Add an extra teaspoon of vanilla per cup of sucralose to cookies, pudding, and custard.
	Sucralose won't activate yeast, so leave at least two teaspoons of sugar in yeast recipes.
	Baked goods made mostly with sucralose won't brown the way sugar-made goods will. To achieve a browned look, spray the items with cooking spray before baking.
Saccharin (Sweet 'N Low, Sweet Twin, Sugar Twin)	Use one cup, or 24 packets, per cup of sugar.
	Don't replace more than half a cup of sugar with saccharin in baked goods.
Aspartame (Nutrasweet, Equal)	Use one cup, or 24 packets, per cup of sugar.
	It loses its sweetness when heated, so use only in recipes that don't require baking, cooking, or otherwise heating.
	Add to recipes after heating. Mix into custards once milk is already hot, or sprinkle on top of foods after baking.
Acesulfame-K (Sunett, Sweet One)	Use 24 packets per cup of sugar.

Some experts do worry about the potential long-term effects of artificial sweeteners, saying undiscovered health problems might not crop up until after decades of use. Some of these substances haven't even been around that long. For this reason, you may want to use them temporarily to wean yourself off of sugary beverages and foods, and avoid long-term use.

Lose weight without really trying

Forget about complicated diets and intense exercise. Getting slim shouldn't seem like rocket science — and with these tricks, it won't.

Take a cold shower. Your body contains a special type of fat that burns calories instead of storing them. It's called brown fat because of its reddish-brown color, and its main job is to keep you warm.

Brown fat doesn't burn calories constantly. It only "turns on" when you get cold. For instance, healthy men who were exposed to cool temperatures for three hours burned 250 more calories than they did at room temperature. The best part is that brown fat actually burns other fats, in the form of triglycerides.

The key is to be cool but not so cold that you shiver. The more the men in this study shivered, the less active their brown fat was.

Build more beneficial brown fat

Brown fat acts like your own fat-burning factory, and now scientists have found a way to create more of it.

Exercise can boost your levels of irisin, a newly discovered hormone that transforms white fat cells, which store extra calories, into brown fat cells, which burn them. Irisin also seems to improve blood sugar and insulin levels.

Exercise may do the trick, but only longer bouts done on a regular basis will raise irisin levels. For example, a 15-minute walk might not help, but a long, fast walk or a long ride on a stationary bike every day might.

Eat the same lunch every day. It might be hard to maintain in the long run, but eating one meal that's the same each day could kick-start your weight loss. It doesn't even need to be a typical "healthy" food.

- In a small study, women who ate macaroni and cheese every day for a week ended up eating 100 fewer calories a day without realizing it.

- A second group of women ate mac and cheese only once a week for five weeks. This became a treat for them, and on their mac-and-cheese days they consumed 30 more calories than usual.

Scientists call it habituation, a fancy word for losing interest in a food you eat often. As a result, you eat less of it. Of course, variety is important for getting all the nutrients your body needs. This trick may not be a long-term fix, but it could be a great way to rev up your weight loss in the short term.

You can also try limiting your food choices. The more options people have about what to eat, the less nutritious the foods they choose and the more they tend to weigh. Cutting back on the variety a little could naturally trim calories from your diet.

Don't share your diet goals. Telling someone how much weight you plan to lose could sabotage your efforts. You'd think that sharing your goal would make you stick to it. But if it's a goal you're really committed to, the opposite seems to happen. Sharing it with someone may make you feel as if you've already achieved something, and you may end up putting less effort into reaching your goal.

You may be able to counteract this effect. Set very specific goals, and say them out loud on a regular basis. For instance, every Saturday you might say, "I am going to lose half a pound by next Friday." Go on to state exactly how you plan to meet that goal, as well as what you'll do if you get off track or stray from your diet.

Stand more, sit less. Exercise isn't the only way to get active. Most people don't work out, but they're probably more active than they think.

- Self-described "couch potatoes" who never exercise still move nine hours a day.

- Homemakers who stand a lot and keep busy spend 12 hours a day in motion.

You may burn a whopping 90 percent of your calories this way, doing the ordinary activities of life. That's 2.5 times more than you burn while sitting. In fact, sitting all day can have a serious impact on weight gain. It can mean the difference between keeping trim and becoming overweight in the course of a single year.

The solution may be simple. Stand up while doing things you'd normally do sitting down. "Many activities like talking on the phone or watching a child's ballgame can be done just as enjoyably upright, and you burn double the number of calories while you're doing it," according to Marc Hamilton, an associate professor of Biomedical Sciences at the University of Missouri-Columbia. Give it a try and see if the pounds start melting away.

Avoid the midmorning munchies. Snacking can do good things for you, like help you eat more fruits and vegetables. But too often it does bad things, especially if you snack when you aren't really hungry.

That's most likely the case when you eat a midmorning snack after having had breakfast. Munching between meals normally helps you eat less at the next one. But munching when you aren't hungry doesn't do that. It simply increases the number of calories you eat in a day.

Out of 123 overweight women on diets, those who ate a midmorning snack lost less weight over the course of a year than women who opted for an afternoon or evening snack, instead. Morning snackers were also more likely to indulge in more than one snack during the day.

Experts say it's not about the time of day you nibble. It's about how long it's been since your last meal. "Our study suggests that snacking may actually help with weight loss if not done too close to another meal, particularly if the snacks are healthy foods that can help you feel full without adding too many calories," says Anne McTiernan, director of the Prevention Center at the Fred Hutchinson Cancer Research Center.

Ask yourself the next time you reach for a bite if you're hungry or just bored, stressed out, or sad. When you do eat something between meals, make it high in fiber but low in calories. "Since women on a weight loss program only have a limited number of calories to spend each day, it is important for them to incorporate nutrient-dense foods that are no more than 200 calories per serving." To that end, McTiernan recommends:

- proteins such as low-fat yogurt, string cheese, or a small handful of nuts.

- nonstarchy vegetables and fresh fruits.

- whole-grain crackers.

- zero-calorie beverages such as water, coffee, and tea.

Stop skipping meals. The same study found that women who skipped meals lost nearly 8 pounds less than other women during one year. That could be because missing one meal makes you more likely to splurge on a rich, high-calorie food later on.

"We also think skipping meals might cluster together with other behaviors," explains McTiernan. "For instance, the lack of time and effort spent on planning and preparing meals may lead a person to skip meals and/or eat out more." Eating out often poses its own problems. "Eating in restaurants usually means less individual control over ingredients and cooking methods, as well as larger portion sizes."

Take steps to make sure you don't have to resort to restaurants or missed meals. Each time you cook soup, stew, or another easy-to-freeze meal, put away at least two servings for a later date. Make this your "emergency fund" and raid it when you don't have the time or energy to whip up a fresh dish.

Diet supplements — do they work?

Most supplements don't do any good, says Melinda Manore, professor of nutrition and exercise sciences at Oregon State University. She reviewed past research and found lots of shoddy science and little effect.

Calcium, green tea, and fiber supplements may have a small impact, helping people lose 3 to 4 pounds, she says. They may help as part of an overall plan.

In the end, however, you can't pop a magic pill and expect to lose weight. "For most people, unless you alter your diet and get daily exercise, no supplement is going to have a big impact," says Manore.

Not to mention the potential side effects. "Some supplements have side effects ranging from the unpleasant, such as bloating and gas, to very serious issues, such as strokes and heart problems," Manore cautions. Stick to safe, proven methods, instead.

7 ways to kick food cravings

Staying strong in the face of temptation is key to winning the battle of the bulge. Arm yourself with this advice to beef up your will and power past the urge to splurge.

Clench your fists. Believe it or not, it can give your willpower a temporary boost. Tightening the muscles in their hands, fingers, calves, or biceps helped people in one study exert more self-control. They were able to ignore tempting foods, endure more pain, choke down an unpleasant medicine, and make tough decisions better than when they were relaxed.

When you exert self-control or call upon your willpower, the muscles in your body involuntarily tighten. Researchers found it can work in reverse, too. Tightening your muscles can briefly strengthen your self-control. This trick only works:

- when you're facing a choice that lines up with your long-term goals. Clenching your muscles might help you pass up dessert at the lunch buffet, but only if one of your goals is to eat healthier or lose weight.

- at the moment of temptation. Wait until you're actively choosing what to eat. Tightening your muscles before you walk into the restaurant won't help. It can backfire and sap your willpower, leaving you vulnerable to cravings.

Sniff a flowery scent. Taking a whiff of jasmine, or any smell that isn't food-related, could take the edge off a chocolate craving. In a slightly heartless experiment, women were shown photos of chocolate to make them long for it. Then they sniffed one of three odors — green apple, jasmine, or plain water. Only the jasmine dampened their desire for the sweet.

Pop a piece of gum. It may quell your craving for sweet stuff. People who chewed sugar-free gum after lunch stayed fuller and craved sweets less.

Smacking on a stick of gum for only 15 minutes an hour helped them eat fewer snacks, especially sweet ones. In all, they ate 40 fewer calories from snacks than when they didn't chew gum. Paula Geiselman, chief of women's health and eating behavior at Pennington Biomedical Research Center, says this simple activity could play a role in "appetite control, reduction of snack cravings, and weight management," albeit a small one. But "even small changes in calories can have an impact in the long term."

Imagine eating candy. Imagining yourself eating something over and over again can help you want it less, and even help you eat less of it when it comes time to indulge. In a series of studies, people were told to imagine themselves doing one of three things:

- inserting 33 quarters into a laundry machine.

- inserting 30 quarters into the machine, then eating three M&M's.

- inserting three quarters and eating 30 M&M's.

Afterward, these same people were allowed to eat as many M&M's as they wanted. Those who had imagined eating 30 of the candies ate the least in real life.

The credit goes to a process known as habituation, where eating the same food over and over leads you to want less of it. "Habituation is one of the fundamental processes that determine how much we consume of a food," explains Joachim Vosgerau, an assistant professor of marketing at Carnegie Mellon University. This research shows that imagining eating it can have the same effect.

The next time you start pining for a particular food, imagine eating it in rich detail. That's key. Simply thinking about a food is not enough. You need to picture yourself eating it in detail, and do it over and over again. Be sure to envision a specific food you're trying to avoid. Thinking about a donut won't help you eat less chocolate cake.

Dream about your favorite place. The next time a hankering for ice cream arises, imagine yourself lying on a sunny beach in Hawaii or fishing on your favorite lake. Anything pleasant will work.

Vividly imagining their favorite activity helped people overcome cravings over the course of four days in one study. The more detail they imagined, the less they yearned for certain foods. Occupying their brains with something meaningless, like saying the alphabet backward, however, didn't help at all.

Eat your Wheaties. Skipping breakfast can make you yearn for junk food. Researchers had 20 people fast overnight and skip breakfast the next day. Then they showed them photographs of high-calorie and low-calorie foods while getting a brain scan. All 20 people came back on a different day, this time having eaten breakfast. Again, researchers showed them photos of food while scanning their brains.

On the day they skipped breakfast, people's brains reacted much more strongly to pictures of rich foods than to low-calorie, healthy foods. Experts say missing this all-important meal seems to bias people toward craving high-calorie foods.

That falls in line with other research showing those who skip breakfast tend to:

- eat 40 percent more sweets.
- drink 55 percent more soft drinks.
- eat fewer vegetables and fruits.

Don't skimp in this area. Enjoy a healthy breakfast every day to get a leg up on weight loss.

Spend more time in bed. Too little sleep can make you crave carbohydrates, says a new study. "In particular, as sleep deprivation increased, self-reported carbohydrate craving also increased," notes Mahmood Siddique, clinical associate professor of medicine at the Robert Wood Johnson Medical School. The sleepier people felt during the day, the more they yearned for high-carb foods.

That's no surprise, since sleep helps regulate your appetite and metabolism. Poor sleep can upset your metabolic system, affect your food choices, and lead to weight gain. Be sure to get plenty of shut-eye, especially if you're on a low-carb eating plan.

The real secret to weight loss

More people are overweight today than hundreds of years ago, and now experts may know why.

Researchers studied the Hadza, a hunter-gatherer tribe in Africa that lives the way people did thousands of years ago. Experts tracked how far they walked and how many calories they burned each day for 11 days.

Surprisingly, the Hadza burned roughly the same calories a day as an average American. That suggests the real culprit behind America's "obesity epidemic" is food. Too much food, and food that's too high in calories. Exercise can help you lose weight and is key for heart health, but this study suggests the key to watching your weight is to watch what you eat.

- Avoid highly processed foods packed with calories but few nutrients.
- Eat plenty of fresh foods prepared at home.
- Steer clear of foods with added sugar and fat.

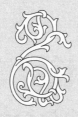

SURE-FIRE WAYS TO DEFEAT DISEASE

Arthritis: super joint soothers

Pill-free ways to kick knee pain

Swallowing pills isn't fun, but you don't know another way to ease your pain. That's about to change. Try these pill-free pain fighters instead.

Strengthen your thighs with leg lifts. Stronger thighs may lower your risk of developing osteoarthritis (OA) in a healthy knee by up to 30 percent. What's more, regular exercise can help reduce pain and stiffness in knees that already have arthritis.

To strengthen your thighs, try this simple leg lift. Lie on your back, and bend one leg enough to comfortably rest your foot on the floor. Raise your other leg so it's level with your other knee. Count to four, and lower your leg to its original position. Do three sets of 10 every day.

Go nuts for fish. To help put out the fire of your joint pain, enjoy foods like salmon, sardines, herring, halibut, trout, light canned tuna, walnuts, and eggs fortified with omega-3. The omega-3 fats in these foods help control the inflammation that causes your arthritis pain. But don't stop there. Most people eat up to 30 times more inflammation-causing foods than inflammation-fighters. So cut back on foods containing omega-6 fats, which encourage inflammation. These include meats, junk food, fried foods, corn oil, safflower oil, soybean oil, and margarine.

Eating nearly equal amounts of omega-6 fats and omega-3 fats every day may help ease the pain of OA and rheumatoid arthritis (RA), experts say. What's more, animal studies suggest a similar diet can prevent, lessen, or delay OA symptoms. Some studies even report that omega-3 fats from fish may reduce joint pain and other arthritis symptoms, helping you cut back on painkillers.

So ease your joint pain by slashing omega-6 fats, and add more fish and other omega-3s to your diet. Just remember, larger fish are more prone to contamination by mercury and other pollutants. To protect yourself, eat a wide variety of fish, and avoid big fish like king mackerel, swordfish, tilefish, shark, wild sturgeon, and bluefish.

Apply a soothing cream. Ask your doctor if you can try a prescription-strength cream or gel in place of your pain-relieving pills. For example, Voltaren and Pennsaid contain prescription doses of the painkiller diclofenac. These topical treatments don't cause stomach irritation, a common side effect with nonsteroidal anti-inflammatory drugs (NSAIDs), like ibuprofen and aspirin, but they may deliver the same amount of medicine to your joints. If you can't use a prescription cream, try a nonprescription cream. Your options include aspirin-derived creams like Aspercreme or Sportscreme; a capsaicin-based cream like Capzasin; or the old standby, BenGay.

Snack on yellow bell peppers. Worsening or new arthritis knee pain may be linked to a shortage of vitamin C. Fortunately, just half of a delicious yellow bell pepper from your super-market has 170 milligrams (mg) of vitamin C — more than a large orange. You need vitamin C for several reasons.

- NSAIDs reduce your vitamin C levels, so you may already be low on vitamin C if you take them for pain.

- Arthritis is less likely to get worse in people who take in high amounts of vitamin C.

- An Australian study of knee MRI scans found that people with a moderate vitamin C intake, 120 to 200 milligrams (mg) a day, had fewer bone marrow lesions — a key source of new arthritis pain.

But the yellow bell pepper doesn't just give you vitamin C. This pepper is also rich in antioxidants, and they may help you avoid suffering from arthritis. When arthritis damages cartilage faster than the cartilage can repair itself, the damaged tissue triggers inflammation and pain. Your body not only needs vitamin C to help repair damaged tissues, like cartilage, it also needs antioxidants to help ease arthritis inflammation.

The next time you want chips and dip, slice a yellow bell pepper into wide, vertical strips and cut each strip in half. It's the perfect curved surface for your favorite dip. Other good sources of vitamin C and antioxidants include strawberries, cranberry juice cocktail, broccoli, pineapple, kiwifruit, orange juice, and oranges.

Fight fire with flavor. A mild variety of onion — the spring onion — can add flavor to your dishes and help protect your body against arthritis at the same time. Spring onions fight arthritis with vitamin C, quercetin, and vitamin K. Quercetin is a phytonutrient that fights inflammation-causing compounds in both OA and RA. For added quercetin, try raw kale, cooked onions, asparagus, cranberries, and radicchio.

Surprisingly, a study of knee X-rays from more than 600 people found more signs of OA in people who didn't get enough vitamin K. If you take blood thinners, like warfarin (Coumadin), talk to your doctor before adding more vitamin K to your diet. Otherwise, boost your vitamin K levels with extra spring onions and leafy greens. You can add spring onions to sandwich fillings, salads, soups, and stir-fries. Not only can those onions help fight arthritis inflammation, they may also help protect you against lung disease and cancer.

Discover the secret painkiller in olive oil

Nature has its own version of the painkiller ibuprofen — oleocanthal, an anti-inflammatory compound in olive oil. It curbs the same inflammation-promoting compounds as ibuprofen and may help fight pain and inflammation like a mini-dose of the popular painkiller. Oleocanthal also cuts excessive production of nitric oxide in your joints, reducing cartilage destruction so arthritis progresses more slowly.

Unfortunately, not all olive oils have oleocanthal. To check whether yours does, sip a little extra virgin olive oil from a teaspoon and swallow. The more it stings the back of your throat, the more oleocanthal it has.

To help ease pain, replace 52 grams of fat in your daily diet with four tablespoons of olive oil. To start, add some to your favorite pasta sauce or make your own vinaigrette salad dressing. Combine 4 tablespoons of olive oil, 2 tablespoons of red wine vinegar, and 1/4 teaspoon of Dijon mustard.

Try a knee brace. Know which brace is right for you. For mild arthritis, the stretchy neoprene or elastic sleeves from your drugstore may be all you need. They compress and warm the knee, provide light support, and gently reduce knee movement. That may be enough to ease or eliminate your pain.

Other braces are available for more severe arthritis, so ask your doctor about your options. For example, if you only have arthritis in one part of your knee, ask your doctor if you are a candidate for an unloader knee brace, and check whether your insurance would cover the cost. In a study funded by the brace maker, all participants reported less pain, stiffness, and disability after six months with an unloader knee brace. Many also needed fewer painkillers.

Eat ginger for pain-free joints. Ginger may make you think of holiday cooking, but using it year round may give you something new to celebrate. Studies show that ginger has anti-inflammatory powers. In fact, it can limit your body's production of prostaglandins and other compounds that cause arthritis inflammation. That's why some experts recommend ginger to ease arthritis pain. Add more ginger to your diet to find out what it can do for you. Slip fresh ginger into stir-fries, soups, cider, and baked goods, and try ginger tea.

For more pain-fighting tactics, see "Surprising ways to manage chronic pain" in the *Super strategies to live long and strong* chapter.

Make friends with ginger

Add ginger to your diet slowly because it can cause heartburn and indigestion. What's more, ginger may not be safe for everyone, so get your doctor's permission before eating large amounts or trying ginger supplements.

7 ways to make living with arthritis easy

Arthritis can make the simplest tasks feel like climbing Mount Everest, but you can turn that mountain back into a molehill. Make traveling, cooking, and other activities more convenient and comfortable with tips and tools like these.

Think ergonomic for relief. Ergonomic tools are clever gadgets that can help you return to cooking and other activities you love. Good examples include a "wide-grip" vegetable peeler with a fat handle or a reach extender rod with a gripper on its far end. You can also find ergonomic garden shears, kitchen knives, and scissors. Just remember to keep the cutting tools sharp so you don't strain your hands, arms, and shoulders while using them.

You can also turn some regular tools into ergonomic tools. For example, wrap rubber bands around your toothbrush handle or wooden spoon handle for a better grip. Wind rubber mesh shelf liner around the handles of kitchen tools, hairbrushes, and other small items to make those handles thicker and easier to grasp. Anchor the liner in place with rubber bands. Buy foam pipe insulation and electrical tape from the home improvement store. Slip the foam around the handles of yard tools, such as rakes or trowels, and secure it with electrical tape.

Work around the problem. Consider labor-saving devices, ideas, or products that do a tough task for you. For example, plan ahead for the next time arthritis prevents you from hand-chopping vegetables for dinner. Buy precut vegetables from the supermarket, invest in an easy-to-operate food processor, or pick up a mini-chopper. Keep an eye out for other labor saving ideas, and you may be surprised at what you can accomplish.

Stretch to fight pain. Stretching may help you reduce pain and stiffness, maintain flexibility and range of motion, improve joint function, and even lubricate your joints. But experts now say static stretching, where you stretch and hold a position, is best saved for after exercise. Dynamic stretching, or stretching while moving, is better for warming up before exercise. Here are two examples of dynamic stretches suggested by the National Arthritis Foundation.

- Arm circles. Stand with your feet apart so each foot is directly below a shoulder. Raise your arms out to the sides at shoulder height, with your palms facing down. Do 20 forward circles followed by 20 backward circles.

- Hip circles. Stand on your right leg, and use a nearby counter or sturdy piece of furniture to help keep your balance. Gently swing your left leg out to your side in a circle. Try to do 20 circles forward and 20 circles backward. Make them as big as you can without causing pain or losing your balance. Turn to stand on your left leg, and do 20 circles in both directions with your right leg.

For additional dynamic stretches, visit *www.arthritistoday.org* and click the Fitness tab. You can also try tai chi, an arthritis-friendly exercise made up of gentle moving stretches. Classes may be available at your church, local senior center, or the Y. Just be sure to get permission from your doctor before you try stretching or any other new exercise.

Try a handheld library. Arthritis can make a favorite book too heavy to hold open. It can even make turning pages difficult. Fortunately, new e-readers are lightweight and make page-turning a breeze. What's more, you can store a whole library of books on one e-reader.

You don't even need to spend money on e-books. You can borrow them from your library or visit the many sources of free e-books online. You won't spend extra money for large print books either. E-readers let you enlarge the font in a regular e-book so it's even bigger than the type in large print books. So consider an e-reader like Amazon's Kindle or the Nook by Barnes & Noble, but make sure you choose one that can download the e-book format your library uses.

Put your luggage on wheels. Carrying large, heavy luggage not only strains your muscles, but your joints, too. Before your next trip, consider buying wheeled luggage or a collapsible, wheeled luggage cart. Make sure your luggage or cart is durable, lightweight, and high quality. This is a worthwhile investment because you can use these for air travel, car travel, and even some in-town travel. For example, use a rolling, carry-on bag instead of an overweight briefcase or purse, or use your luggage cart to transport heavy or unwieldy items from one room to another.

Choose the right chair. Be picky when you replace your favorite easy chair. Sit in the chair before you buy it, and notice whether your feet are flat on the floor. You don't want a chair that is too high or too low. Also, make sure soft cushioning doesn't let you sink too low, or you may struggle to rise out of the chair.

Test the armrests to be certain they are sturdy and can assist you in sitting down and getting up. Make sure the armrest is high enough to support your elbows when you sit, but not uncomfortably high.

Get a rubdown. You may wonder how massage could have any effect on arthritis. But, according to research, massage can:

- trigger the release of endorphins, your body's natural painkillers.

- loosen muscles and other tissues tightened by arthritis, and improve range of motion.

- lower production of substance P, a neurotransmitter linked to pain.

- improve pain, stiffness, hand strength, walking ability, and joint performance.

Massage is not right for everyone, so ask your doctor if it's safe for you before you try it. Find out whether your insurance covers massage, too. If it does, ask your doctor or physical therapist for a referral to a certified massage therapist. Make sure the therapist knows about your arthritis and any medications you take and is willing to do a gentle or moderate massage. Then just relax and enjoy being pampered.

Find ergonomic products that really work

You've heard about helpful products like easy-to-open medicine bottles, scissors that spring open after each cut, arthritis-friendly resealable food-storage bags, and neck-cradling pillows. But you wonder if they really help prevent pain and make life easier. To be sure you get the advantages you pay for, look for the Arthritis Foundation's Ease-of-Use Commendation logo.

Earning the logo is tough. Scientists at Atlanta's Georgia Tech Research Institute test whether each product and its packaging meet basic ease-of-use requirements, and whether they remain easy to use in various common situations. In fact, people with moderate-to-severe arthritis also test the product. Products that pass the tests can display the Ease-of-Use Commendation logo on their packages. For a list of products that have earned this logo, visit *www.arthritis.org.*

5 arthritis myths you should know about

Every week the TV show Mythbusters puts rumors, TV and movie cliches, or news stories to the test. They have checked everything from whether milk can douse the fire of hot peppers to whether a person can dodge a bullet. If they were to dedicate a show to myths about arthritis, they might test claims like these.

Claim: The best shoes for arthritis are athletic shoes with built-in support. Stiff, padded shoes may feel like solid foot protection, but remember this. The amount of stress a shoe puts on your knee joint may affect your odds of knee arthritis and determine how quickly arthritis gets worse. A recent study found that foot-stabilizing athletic shoes and cushioned feet-protecting clogs caused more knee stress in people with knee arthritis than a flat, flexible walking shoe. The researchers suggest flat, flexible shoes cause less stress because they mimic walking barefoot.

Of course, the study only examined a few people and a few types of shoes, so more research is needed. For example, some experts say athletic shoes that control the foot's movement or stability may still be good for some people with various kinds of arthritis, including knee arthritis. To learn about the latest recommendations, ask your doctor what kind of shoes are best for you.

Claim: Drinking coffee causes gout. Drinking coffee after dinner may keep you up at night, but it won't give you gout. In fact, research suggests regular or decaffeinated coffee may reduce your risk of gout. One recent study found that women who drank four or more cups of coffee daily had 57 percent less risk of gout than women who drank no coffee. Drinking coffee every day protects men from gout, too. Coffee may help because it lowers your blood levels of uric acid, which can build up and cause gout. Researchers suspect chlorogenic acid, an antioxidant found in coffee, may be the reason why.

Claim: All exercise is good for arthritis. Jogging, football, and full-court basketball involve running, jumping, and other high-impact exercise that can make your joints worse. Replace joint-jarring exercise with low-impact choices like swimming, walking, yoga, tai chi, cycling, or water aerobics. Yet even these exercises aren't foolproof. To help avoid joint damage, reduce pain and stiffness, and improve your range of motion, remember these tips.

- Ask your doctor what exercises are safe for you. If pain and inflammation are a problem, ask him how to get them under control before you begin a new workout or exercise program.

- Start slowly and gradually increase the length and intensity of your exercise.

- Warm up with gentle, range-of-motion exercises before working out.

- Rotate among different kinds of low-impact exercises to avoid strain.

- Stop exercising immediately if you experience moderate or severe pain. If joint pain appears after a workout, shorten future workouts that affect that joint or lower their intensity.

Claim: Losing weight doesn't ease arthritis pain as much as painkillers. According to a survey of 1 million people, those who were overweight reported 20 percent higher rates of pain than people with a normal BMI — or body mass index. Obese people reported pain rates at least 68 percent higher. Yet extra load on your lower limbs may not be the only cause of pain, because obesity has also been linked to developing arthritis in hands.

This may happen because obesity creates extra fat cells. Recent research suggests those cells produce hormones that rev up inflammation in your body and may contribute to arthritis pain. Fortunately, losing even small amounts of weight can make a surprising difference, especially if you have knee arthritis. If you are overweight, Johns Hopkins researchers say, losing just 15 pounds may ease your pain more than popular painkillers. What's more, losing 1 pound of weight removes 4 pounds of stress on your knees.

Claim: All glucosamine supplements are the same. A 2005 review of studies found that glucosamine sulfate slowed the progress of arthritis and reduced pain, but glucosamine hydrochloride performed no better than placebo pills. More research is needed, so talk with your doctor before you try glucosamine sulfate. If she says yes, read labels carefully before you buy. Keep in mind it could be at least six weeks before you see results. Because most glucosamine comes from shellfish, don't take glucosamine supplements if you are allergic to shellfish.

Beware the flop in flip-flops

You are thinking about buying some cute flip-flops, especially since research suggests flip-flops are as good for your knees as going barefoot. Unfortunately, these shoes raise your risk of falling. In fact, the United Kingdom's National Health Service reportedly spends millions every year on falls and other injuries involving flip-flops. Experts say you should limit wearing flip-flops to short periods when you only expect to walk on flat surfaces.

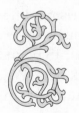

Cancer: smart ways to keep it at bay

5 cancer-causing foods to avoid at all costs

When it comes to cancer protection, sometimes what you don't eat is just as important as what you do eat. Keep these cancer-causing foods in mind the next time you go to the supermarket or out to dinner.

Watch out for processed meats. Hot dogs, bologna, and other processed meats contain nitrites and nitrates to stop bacteria from growing and keep it looking fresh. Unfortunately, too much of these substances may raise your risk of developing colorectal and stomach cancers, among others.

Researchers found that people who eat the most nitrites and nitrates from processed meats and get lots of the compounds from other foods, like vegetables and fruits, have up to a 29-percent higher risk of bladder cancer. That's compared to people who eat the least amount of nitrites.

The problem with nitrites and nitrates is still being studied, but it's possible your body converts them to potentially cancer-causing compounds called nitrosamines. So ditch the cold cuts, and enjoy leftover roasted turkey on your sandwiches instead.

Head off cancer with one common fruit

Add some lemon or lemon peel to your tea, and you may ward off at least 11 kinds of cancer.

Researchers in Japan found that people who ate more citrus fruits had lower rates of nearly a dozen types of cancer over the next nine years. Oranges, tangerines, lemons, limes, and grapefruits were included on the list. Those with the lowest risk of cancer also drank at least one cup of green tea daily.

Cancer of the liver, breast, uterus, prostate, esophagus, pancreas, stomach, colorectum, lung, kidney, and bladder were among the types reduced by people eating citrus and drinking tea. Experts suspect natural plant chemicals in citrus, including flavonoids, vitamins, naringenin, and d-limonene, may provide the anti-cancer power.

Even citrus peel packs a punch. A study in Arizona — the land of sunshine — found that people who drank more black tea with citrus peel had lower rates of skin cancer.

Say no to charred meat. Of course, you have to cook meat long enough to kill dangerous bacteria, but don't overdo it. Those black lines on steak from the grill mean it's contaminated with cancer-causing compounds like heterocyclic amines (HCAs) and polycyclic aromatic hydrocarbons (PAHs).

These killer compounds form when meat is cooked at high temperatures, like when grilling or broiling. They're known to cause DNA changes in animals, and they're suspected of causing colorectal cancer in people who eat a lot of meat.

259

You can cut your risk by cooking meat differently. Pick steaming, poaching, stewing, or microwaving over grilling. It's also a good idea to wrap meat in tin foil with holes poked in it before grilling to let fat drip out, but limit the smoke that gets onto the meat. And marinating meat may also cut your exposure to HCAs.

Simply eating more meat of all kinds seems to raise your risk of a variety of cancers.

- One study showed that men who eat more well-done grilled and barbecued meat — along with more red meat and processed meat altogether — raise their risk of suffering an aggressive form of prostate cancer.

- Australian researchers found that women who ate the most meat and fat were more likely to develop ovarian cancer than those who ate less.

- Another study showed that middle-aged people who eat the most red meat have a 19-percent higher risk of some types of kidney cancer.

Skip salt-cured and pickled foods. The American Cancer Society warns that people who eat large amounts of food preserved by salting and pickling may have a higher risk of stomach, throat, and nasopharyngeal cancers. These foods may not be staples in the United States, but they are in other parts of the world.

Researchers looked at Japanese immigrants in Brazil and the United States to see how changing diets might affect their cancer risk. Their traditional diets in Japan included lots of pickled vegetables, salted fish and roe, and highly salted foods like miso soup. Men who continued eating this traditional diet had higher rates of gastric cancer.

The dangers may be related to the fact that a higher intake of salted food often goes along with the risk of *Helicobacter pylori* infection. These bacteria, which can live in your stomach, are also a risk factor for stomach cancer.

The good news, as the researchers point out, is that as people in Japan are turning to more fresh fruits and vegetables rather than those traditional staples, their risk of gastric cancer drops.

Limit French fries and baked goods. These tasty treats may be your favorite part of the meal, but they can be loaded with acrylamides. These natural compounds form during the browning process of high-carb foods like cereals, bread, chips, and French fries. Scientists think they increase inflammation in your body and raise your risk of heart disease.

Acrylamides may also raise your risk of endometrial cancer and possibly ovarian cancer. Researchers looked at data from the Nurses' Health Study, which followed more than 120,000 women for 26 years. They checked to see what the women had been eating over that time and how many developed cancers of the breast, ovaries, and endometrium, or lining of the uterus.

Turns out women who ate more foods with acrylamides were not at any greater risk for developing breast cancer. But they did have a higher risk of endometrial cancer and a slightly higher risk for ovarian cancer.

You can limit your exposure by cooking smart. Cut potatoes into thicker pieces, and blanch them before making fries. And in general, limit the amount of golden-brown fries and baked goods you eat.

Control your alcohol intake. The American Cancer Society says alcohol raises your risk of certain cancers — especially if you

261

drink more than two drinks daily for men and more than one drink for women.

Tons of research over the years has shown how drinking alcohol in excess can raise your risk of cancer, including oral and pharyngeal cancer, liver cancer, breast cancer, colorectal cancer, and pancreatic cancer. Generally speaking, the more you drink, the greater your risk. For example, a habit of four or more drinks a day is associated with a fivefold increase in your risk of developing oral, pharyngeal, and esophageal cancer.

But there may be a reason for women to continue enjoying a glass of red wine. New research hints that red wine contains aromatase inhibitors, natural compounds that help lower the level of estrogen in your body, a change that can reduce your risk of breast cancer.

Warning — tippling ups risk of stroke

In spite of its effect on cancer risk, an occasional alcoholic beverage may have long-term benefits for your heart. In the short-term, beware. Your stroke risk doubles in the hour after you drink alcohol.

Researchers at three different medical centers surveyed people who had suffered stroke to find out whether they drank any alcohol during the time before the stroke. They found the risk of ischemic stroke rose to be 2.3 times higher in the hour after drinking as little as one alcoholic beverage. Ischemic strokes occur when blood flow to brain cells is blocked.

Stroke risk returned to normal by the time three hours had passed. All types of alcohol had an effect, from beer and wine to hard liquor.

Experts aren't sure why stroke risk increases, but they think it may be related to the fact that your blood pressure rises temporarily when you drink alcohol.

"If you were to have a glass of wine with dinner, you may want to consider a glass of red," says study co-author Chrisandra Shufelt, MD. "Switching may shift your risk."

Other research has pointed out that people who drink in moderation may cut their risk of heart disease and heart attack, lower their cholesterol, and reduce stroke risk. But fighting heart disease is not a good reason to start drinking alcohol.

Cancer protection in 30 minutes a day

Protecting yourself from cancer is easier than you think. Just a few minutes every day will help cut your risk.

Eat your veggies. A study of more than 2,700 men revealed that more fiber in their diets meant less chance of prostate cancer. But listen up before you grab your cereal bowl — the effective fiber came from vegetables, especially crucifers like broccoli.

Researchers in a study in Italy questioned 2,745 men about their eating habits over the previous two years and discovered that those with the lowest risk of prostate cancer had been eating the most vegetables.

Another study in Seattle looked at the diets of men younger than 65 years, finding that those who eat more cruciferous vegetables each week have a lower risk of prostate cancer. Men who eat 28 servings of vegetables a week — about four servings a day — had a 35-percent lower risk of prostate cancer compared to men who ate fewer than 14 servings each week.

And women can also benefit from vegetable fiber, as shown by a study of Chinese women living in Singapore. Middle-age women were able to cut their risk of breast cancer by eating more cabbage, bok choy, kale, and broccoli, among other vegetables and fruits.

Experts aren't sure why vegetable fiber protects against cancer. They suspect it may be related to how some fibers delay starch absorption in your intestines, thus cutting the glycemic load of the food you eat. To get your four servings a day, learn to love these fiber-filled favorites.

- Brussels sprouts, with 3 grams (g) fiber in one-half cup

- broccoli, with 1 g fiber in one-half cup

- cauliflower, with 2 g fiber in one-half cup

- cabbage, with 2 g fiber in one-half cup

Keep vitamin A in balance. Taking a vitamin A supplement may help protect you from melanoma, the most deadly but least common form of skin cancer, but you don't want to overdo it.

Researchers found that people who took a daily vitamin A supplement for 10 years were 60 percent less likely to develop melanoma than those who skipped it.

Women in the study seemed to be more protected by vitamin A than men, possibly because men may be more susceptible to skin damage from UV radiation.

But too much of this common vitamin can weaken your bones and cause joint pain. Experts say getting more than 5,000 to 10,000 international units (IU) a day of vitamin A can raise your risk of osteoporosis and breaking a hip. The danger is even greater for people who don't get enough vitamin D, since vitamin A can suppress the activity of vitamin D in your body.

Other symptoms of excess vitamin A include muscle and joint pain, headache, fatigue, dry skin and lips, nausea, and hair loss. Getting vitamin A from foods like carrots and sweet potatoes is usually considered safe, but supplements can give you too much at once.

For more information on getting the right amount of vitamin A, see "When vitamins kill" in the *Super strategies to live long and strong* chapter.

Take a walk. As little as one hour each week of exercise — something as easy as walking — can stave off some cancers. One study found activity can cut your risk of colon polyps, which sometimes lead to colon cancer. The effect was strongest for people who were overweight.

Other research found that men diagnosed with prostate cancer who take brisk walks have less chance of seeing their cancer progress. They got the most benefit from walking at least 3 miles per hour, and the effect was strongest when they walked three hours a week or more. You can break up the activity into two walks of 15 minutes each a day, so it's not a huge time commitment.

Stacey Kenfield, a researcher at Harvard School of Public Health and lead author of the study, pointed out the benefits of even minor amounts of exercise.

"We observed benefits at very attainable levels of activity and our results suggest that men with prostate cancer should do some physical activity for their overall health, even if it is a small amount, such as 15 minutes of activity per day of walking, jogging, biking or gardening," said Kenfield.

If you get a bit sore as you start being active, consider taking aspirin to ease your pain. As the accompanying feature shows, aspirin may also help protect you from cancer.

Aspirin may be anti-cancer 'wonder drug'

Taking a daily aspirin to keep your heart healthy is old news. Your doctor may already have you on daily baby aspirin therapy to prevent a heart attack or stroke. But you may also be reaping a bonus from that amazing little pill — protection from certain cancers.

Digestive cancers are aspirin's biggest targets. Hundreds of studies between 1950 and 2011 tracked how aspirin affects your body. Researchers analyzed this data, following some people for 20 years to check for cancer.

The strongest evidence was related to aspirin and colon cancer, along with other cancers that affect your digestive system, such as stomach and esophageal cancer. Regular use of aspirin was associated with a lower risk of colorectal cancer, and it also seemed to slow the spread of colon cancer to other organs in your body. That might make it a good treatment for those who already have cancer.

Other research has shown aspirin may help keep you safe from cancers of the lungs, breast, and prostate. Along with preventing tumor growth, aspirin may cut your risk of dying of cancer by 37 percent if you take it for five years or more.

Even the experts don't know just how aspirin affects cancer risk. It may be because aspirin blocks the COX-2 enzyme, which raises inflammation in your body and is abundant in tumors. Or it could be connected to aspirin's effects on platelet function in your body.

Before you start taking daily aspirin to sidestep cancer, talk to your doctor about the possible benefits and risks, which include bleeding ulcer and hemorrhagic stroke.

7 facts you didn't know about breast cancer

You know when you should schedule a mammogram and how to do a lump check, and you support those pink ribbon groups. But there's more to breast cancer than scans and fund-raising. Learn seven new tidbits about how to avoid and deal with this common killer.

More hot flashes mean a lower risk. If you suffered more than your friends from the effects of menopause — hot flashes, sleepless nights, vaginal dryness — you can thank your lucky stars in one respect. It's a sign you may have a lower risk of breast cancer.

Researchers talked to more than 1,000 women ages 55 to 74 who had gone through menopause, asking about their symptoms. They found that women who suffered the typical side effects of the change of life were less likely to develop one of two common forms of breast cancer later — invasive ductal carcinoma and invasive lobular carcinoma. Women who had no menopausal symptoms had a higher risk of cancer.

And the worse your menopausal symptoms, the better, since stronger hot flashes meant an even lower cancer risk. The protection is likely due to the declining levels of estrogen in your body that trigger hot flashes.

Sleep is not just for your beauty. It's also key to avoiding the most aggressive forms of breast cancer. A new study finds lack of sleep may increase your risk of developing a more aggressive breast cancer along with the risk of cancer recurrence.

Researchers in Cleveland found that postmenopausal women diagnosed with breast cancer had a greater chance of aggressive breast cancer if they got six hours of sleep or less each night during the previous two years. Sleep-deprived women were also more likely to suffer from cancer recurrence.

Lead author Cheryl Thompson, Ph.D., points out the importance of getting enough sleep. "This is the first study to suggest that women who routinely sleep fewer hours may develop more aggressive breast cancers compared with women who sleep longer hours," she says.

Because the study was done on postmenopausal women, it's not known whether your premenopausal breast cancer risk may also be affected by sleep. Better get some rest, just to be sure.

High-tech way to detect breast cancer

Ask about a high-tech option if you and your doctor agree you need a mammogram to check for signs of breast cancer.

Researchers teamed up with a mammography clinic that was switching from using traditional film screening to digital mammography. They found that more breast cancers were located when the new technique was used. The detection rate rose from 4.1 to 7.9 tumors for every 1,000 women screened.

The researchers believe digital mammograms provide more details than can be seen with film. Another benefit of choosing digital is that you are exposed to less radiation than from a conventional mammogram.

When you go digital, be sure your results are read by a radiologist and not by a computer. Machine-read digital mammograms are more likely to lead to false positive results.

Staying healthy can cut your risk. It's a fact that nearly one-third of all cancer deaths are related to being overweight and sedentary. Now experts in Sweden warn that having diabetes or being obese when you get older may be a sign you're at greater risk of breast cancer.

They evaluated health data from some 1.5 million people in that country, relating chronic conditions with breast cancer risk. Two major findings stood out.

- Obesity in women older than 60 years increased their risk of breast cancer by 55 percent.

- Women who had been diagnosed with diabetes at least four years earlier were at 37-percent higher risk of breast cancer.

More research is needed to see if the results hold true for other populations. But it's known that excess weight raises the amount of estrogen fat cells release to circulate in your body, which ups your risk of breast cancer.

Exercise may help you avoid breast cancer. Researchers looked at results of the Long Island Breast Cancer Study Project, which followed more than 3,000 women, half with breast cancer and half without. They wanted to see which of these women exercised.

They found that women who exercised during their reproductive years and after menopause had a lower risk of developing breast cancer. Those who got active between 10 and 19 hours each week had the greatest protection, with a 30-percent lower risk. Protection seemed greatest against hormone receptor positive breast cancer — ER or PR positive — the most common type among American women.

Exercise was beneficial at all levels of intensity, not only sprint workouts and the like. But 10 to 19 hours a week comes to an average of two hours a day. That's not peanuts, so find an activity you really enjoy. Then stick with it, and build up some protection.

Baking soda may be drink of the future

Researchers suspect drinking baking soda dissolved in water may keep breast cancer from spreading. Now they can test this idea. A government grant of $2 million will let University of Arizona researchers use magnetic resonance imaging (MRI) to check the acidity of a tumor.

Growing tumors produce lactic acid — the same substance that makes muscles sore during exercise. When it comes from a tumor, the lactic acid kills healthy tissue to let the tumor grow. Some cancer drugs don't work at a low, or acidic, pH. But raising the tumor's pH might make the drugs more effective.

Previous research showed that when cancerous mice drank a mixture of water and baking soda, they had a higher pH around their tumors and less cancer spreading to other organs. They also lived longer than mice who drank plain water.

Experts are waiting for results of the Arizona study before trying it on people.

One in 1,000 men get breast cancer. Men in the United States suffered from about 2,190 new cases of invasive breast cancer in 2012. Roughly 410 men would die from the disease.

Some risk factors for breast cancer are the same for men as for women, such as a family history, obesity, and advancing age. But others are specific to men, including an undescended testicle and certain genetic conditions.

The American Cancer Society says even men should be aware of the warning signs. See a doctor if you experience any of these symptoms.

- new lump in breast

- skin dimpling or puckering

- nipple retraction

- scaling or redness of breast skin

- nipple discharge

Treatment side effects can go on and on. Of course, if you have breast cancer you have to go through the treatment that's right for you. But chemotherapy, radiation, and major surgery come with a price, in terms of side effects. New research shows some effects can last for years.

Women in Australia who were treated for breast cancer were followed for six years. More than 60 percent of the women still suffered from at least one negative side effect after all those years.

Side effects included skin problems from radiation, postsurgical complications like infections, weight gain, and fatigue. Some women reported upper-body symptoms such as pain, numbness, stiffness, and limited range of motion in their arms. Lymphedema, or painful swelling of the arms from excess fluid, was also a problem.

Many of these symptoms can be improved with the right rehabilitation, so the researchers pointed out the need to offer help to women long after their cancer treatment is done.

Some older women can skip radiation treatment. Research shows that not all women older than 70 years benefit from getting radiation therapy after breast cancer surgery. The particular stage of cancer may help determine whether it's worth it.

A study of older women who had a mastectomy for invasive breast cancer identified the women as either low risk, medium risk, or high risk for recurrence. Researchers followed the women for more than six years to see how they fared from treatment. Only women in the high-risk group benefited from getting radiation treatment after their mastectomies in terms of longer survival. Those in the other groups did not benefit from radiation.

Radiation therapy has its drawbacks, including skin irritation, fatigue, and pain, as well as extra cost and inconvenience.

Know which tests to avoid and to consider

Doctors can do many different tests and scans, looking for problems in every part of your body. Some of these tests help save lives by finding cancers in time to treat and even cure them. But finding more problems doesn't always mean better health. In some cases, tests can find oddities in your body that aren't really a problem — and the tests can have health risks.

Think twice before you schedule these tests. Evidence of their usefulness is shaky in certain situations.

PSA blood test with no symptoms or risk factors. Too much prostate-specific antigen (PSA) in your blood isn't always a sign of prostate cancer. Only a biopsy can determine if you have cancer. Risks of having a biopsy or other treatments include impotence, incontinence, heart attack, and even death. In contrast, a small, slow-growing prostate tumor may never cause a problem.

It's a tricky issue, but the American Society of Clinical Oncology says men should ask their doctors whether they need a PSA test if they are not expected to live longer than 10 years. This organization does not give specific age recommendations, but it says to consider other health conditions that affect your risk.

Even more surprising, the U.S. Preventive Services Task Force (USPSTF) sees no value in screening men of any age who have no symptoms.

Pap smear after age 65. The USPSTF says you don't need to have Pap tests after age 65 to screen for cervical cancer if you've had three normal tests in a row. Previous recommendations suggested stopping at age 70.

New recommendations say healthy women between 21 and 65 years old can have the test every three years.

Dental X-rays every year. Researchers found that people who have more bitewing dental X-rays — annually or more often — have a higher risk of intracranial meningioma, a type of brain tumor. Most X-rays in the study were done in years past, when machines used more radiation than they do now.

But it's best to question your dentist about the diagnostic benefit of an X-ray. And see about wearing a thyroid guard or shield while having an X-ray. This special lead collar can protect your delicate thyroid from radiation.

On the other hand, don't miss these important tests. Experts say they are well worth having done, and they could save your life.

Colonoscopy — observe the guidelines. This test does more than just find cancer — it lets doctors remove colon polyps that could turn into cancer later.

You may not relish the thought of having a colonoscopy, but it's a test that can save your life. The USPSTF recommends most people get one every 10 years from age 50 to 75. Follow these guidelines:

- Have your colonoscopy done by a gastroenterologist rather than by a surgeon or primary care doctor. Research shows older folks who had their tests done by gastroenterologists — who get extra training in the procedure — were less likely to die of colon cancer.

- Prep correctly for the procedure. One study found colonoscopies done without good preparation tend to miss polyps, possibly leading to a repeat procedure in less than three years.

Mammogram — follow recommendations. There's been lots of debate over what age and how often to have a mammogram to screen for breast cancer. Don't make that your excuse to skip the test altogether.

The American College of Obstetricians and Gynecologists recommends that women age 50 and older have a screening mammogram every year. In contrast, the USPSTF says women 50 to 74 years old should get one every two years.

That advice changes if you're at higher risk due to a strong family history of breast cancer, like having a mutation in the BRCA1 or BRCA2 genes, or a history of chest radiation. Then a mammogram is recommended more often.

Transvaginal ultrasound if you have symptoms. This test helps determine the thickness of the uterine wall to find cancer. A technician inserts a special ultrasound probe into the vagina, capturing images of the uterine wall.

There's a certain risk of false positive results, since some women show a thick uterine wall even without having cancer. But the test is noninvasive, so experts recommend having it done if you have symptoms of uterine cancer, such as abnormal bleeding or other unusual discharge.

Heart imaging test not without cancer risks

You may think screening tests are safe, but that's not always the case. A test to check for clogged arteries exposes you to as much radiation as 51 mammograms or 309 chest X-rays. That's why you should ask your doctor whether you really need CT angiography to diagnose a heart problem.

Researchers found that one of every 270 women who underwent CT angiography at age 40 developed cancer later. Many doctors prefer using traditional angiography to view the state of your arteries, since this test uses less radiation. It's also cheaper and possibly more accurate than CT angiography.

The American Heart Association recommends against having a heart-imaging study involving radiation if you have no chest pain or other symptoms of heart disease. Ask your doctor what test is best, and keep a record of your test results to avoid repeat procedures.

Latest tips to battle prostate cancer

Prostate cancer is the most commonly found cancer in men, with about one in six men expected to be diagnosed in their lifetimes. Keep up with current research so you can stay safe from this all-too-familiar killer.

Think twice before you crack an egg. Researchers wanted to find out whether eating red meat, chicken, or eggs could raise your risk of prostate cancer. They followed more than 27,000 men from 1994 to 2008, surveying what they ate and whether they were diagnosed with prostate cancer.

Turns out only egg consumption had any link to prostate cancer. Men who ate at least two and one-half eggs a week had an 81-percent higher risk of deadly prostate cancer than men who ate less than half an egg each week. Eating meat and poultry didn't have any effect.

The experts don't know why eggs might raise your risk, but they suspect it's either the choline or the cholesterol in eggs. Both of these natural substances have been shown to be abundant in the blood of men with prostate cancer.

An earlier study showed that men with the highest choline levels had a 48-percent greater risk of prostate cancer than men with the lowest levels. Cancer cells use lots of choline, an essential nutrient. Cancerous prostate cells, in particular, use it especially quickly.

Cancer cells hamper your body's ability to keep cholesterol in balance. High levels of cholesterol may encourage the production of androgens — male sex hormones — and other changes that encourage prostate tumor growth.

Enjoy exotic spice's many health benefits. It's old news that curcumin, the spice that makes curry powder yellow, can protect your brain from age-related changes. That's because curcumin works as an anti-inflammatory in your body.

But new research shows how eating more curry may help you steer clear of prostate cancer. One study found that curcumin:

- kept prostate cancer cells from multiplying.

- prevented them from spreading to other areas.

- blocked inflammation, keeping cancer from developing in the first place and triggering existing cancer cells to die off.

These results show curcumin might prevent, and one day even treat, prostate cancer. Experts say it might work well alongside conventional cancer treatments.

Curcumin dissolves in fat but not in water, and your body doesn't absorb it well in the intestines. When adding curry spice to your food, remember that black pepper and a bit of oil help your body absorb curcumin.

Ask about more focus in treatment. High-intensity focused ultrasound (HIFU) treats prostate tumors as small as a grain of rice without damaging surrounding healthy cells. It does this by focusing heat directly onto cancerous cells, so there's little risk of side effects.

Current standard treatments for prostate tumors — surgery and radiation therapy — carry a big risk of impotence and incontinence. That's why some men are reluctant to have small tumors treated.

But a small study on HIFU showed it offered targeted treatment with no side effects in nine of 10 men treated. After a year, during which a few men were retreated with more HIFU, 39 of 41 men in the study were free of cancer. And 95 percent of them had no lasting urinary or sexual side effects.

HIFU treatment is not yet approved by the Food and Drug Administration (FDA) in the United States, but it may be available soon.

Be wary of can-do drugs. There's new information on possible benefits and risks of drugs like finasteride (Proscar) and dutasteride (Avodart). You may already be taking one of these 5-alpha-reductase inhibitors for benign prostatic hyperplasia (BPH). Some research indicates they may help protect against prostate cancer, but other studies say it increases your risk.

The issue is complicated. Drugs in this class seem to slow down prostate enlargement, or BPH, which is good. And some research shows they can also slow the growth of low-grade prostate tumors — those with a Gleason score of 6 or less. These tumors are not likely to be deadly.

But other research hints that 5-alpha reductase inhibitors may encourage the growth of higher-grade, or more deadly, prostate tumors with higher Gleason scores.

Talk to your doctor if you are already taking one of these drugs for BPH. You can decide together if it may be raising or lowering your risk of prostate cancer.

Protect your gut from radiation

Taking probiotics before a radiation treatment may protect your intestines from damage.

Radiation therapy is used to treat cancerous tumors of the bladder and other abdominal organs. But it can kill healthy cells in the process, damaging the lining of your small intestines and bringing on bouts of severe diarrhea. Sometimes it's so bad, a cancer patient may have to reduce or end radiation treatment.

The same probiotics you can take to keep powerful antibiotics from ravaging your body's natural flora may help. Probiotics can replenish the helpful microorganisms your body needs to function properly.

Research in mice found the common probiotic *Lactobacillus rhamnosus GG* (LGG) can protect the intestinal lining when it's taken before radiation treatment. LGG is similar to the natural bacteria found in yogurt, and it's already available in pill form. What's more, the study used relatively small doses. But experts say more information is needed before LGG treatment is used in people.

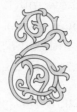

Diabetes: fast fixes for blood sugar problems

Surefire ways to sidestep sugar spikes

After scoring a touchdown, a football player might spike the ball in triumph. Unlike a touchdown, a spike in blood sugar is nothing to celebrate. Concentrated sources of sugar, such as soda or candy, and refined white starch, like white bread or rice, can cause your blood sugar to rapidly skyrocket. Here's how to avoid these unhealthy fluctuations in blood sugar.

Find the right fruit. Love to eat fruits, but worried about sugar spikes? Try the fabulous fruit that has no effect on your blood sugar but will lower cholesterol — the kiwi. Named for the hairy, flightless national bird of New Zealand, the kiwi has a hairy, dull-brown skin. Inside, it sports emerald green flesh, with rows of black, edible seeds. Officially known as kiwifruit, this unusual fruit tastes like a blend of strawberry, pineapple, and sweet melon.

One large kiwifruit provides 3 grams of fiber, which helps lower cholesterol and slows the absorption of sugar into the bloodstream. It also boasts a very low glycemic load (GL) of 4. Glycemic load measures how much a serving of food is likely to increase your blood sugar levels. You calculate it by multiplying a food's glycemic index (GI), as a percentage, by the number of net carbohydrates in a given serving.

You can also eat a fresh fig, which gives you 2 grams of fiber and has a GL of 4. Other good choices for people with diabetes include high-fiber fruits like apples, pears, apricots, blueberries, strawberries, pomegranates, and avocados.

Stir in some psyllium. Another way to add fiber to your diet is by adding psyllium to your beverages. Stir this powder into your orange juice before meals, and reduce the after-eating jump in blood glucose. As a bonus, it also helps improve your heart health and combats constipation.

Studies show that, for people with diabetes, psyllium lowers blood sugar after eating a meal. It also lowers cholesterol in people with diabetes who have high cholesterol. You may lower total cholesterol by 9 percent and LDL cholesterol by 13 percent.

To reap these benefits, aim for 15 grams of psyllium a day, taken in three divided doses. Just stir the powder into an 8-ounce beverage, like fruit juice or water, at mealtimes. But make sure to monitor your blood sugar levels, so they don't drop too low. If you take diabetes medication, you may need to lower your dose when taking psyllium.

Of course, psyllium — most commonly sold under the brand name Metamucil — is best known for its work as a bulk-forming laxative. So if you're dealing with constipation, psyllium can also help get your bowels moving again.

Count on chromium. Battling type 2 diabetes? Make sure you eat plenty of whole grains, asparagus, nuts, and liver. They contain chromium, a workhorse nutrient that shuttles excess sugar out of your bloodstream and into your cells.

Because chromium helps regulate glucose in the blood, it should prevent sugar spikes. This important mineral works by teaming up with insulin to help it unlock the "door" to the cell membrane so glucose in your bloodstream can enter the cell.

Evidence suggests that chromium supplements may improve blood sugar control in people with diabetes. They may even help people with insulin resistance, or an impaired response to insulin, and mildly high blood sugar levels. Talk to your doctor to determine the right type of chromium supplement and the proper dosage.

But you can also get chromium from your diet. The most concentrated sources of chromium are brewer's yeast and calf liver. Other good food sources include whole grains, beer, and cheese. You can also find chromium in beef, chicken, dairy products, eggs, seafood, mushrooms, asparagus, potatoes with skin, prunes, nuts, and fresh fruit, especially apples with skin.

Sweeten with stevia. Among low-calorie sweeteners, stevia may provide the lowest risk of sugar spikes. It can also help you cut calories without feeling hungry.

In one study, 19 lean and 12 obese people received an appetizer, or "preload," of tea, crackers, and cream cheese sweetened with either stevia, aspartame, or sucrose 20 minutes before lunch and dinner. Over three test days, each person tried each sweetener without knowing its identity.

While they could eat as much or as little of each meal as they wanted, it turns out they didn't overcompensate for the low-calorie sweeteners by eating more later. And they felt just as full as when they ate the high-calorie sucrose preload.

Better yet, blood tests showed that stevia reduced glucose levels after eating compared to sucrose and lowered insulin levels compared to both aspartame and sucrose. These results suggest that stevia may help with glucose regulation.

5 reasons to make room for mushrooms

While you're changing your diet for the better, don't forget about the humble mushroom. The Chinese called this edible fungus the "elixir of life" — and no wonder. Research finds it could boost your immune system, reduce inflammation, lower blood sugar, and help prevent blood clots, and they may even fight certain types of tumors.

Researchers in Australia found that simple white button mushrooms lowered blood sugar and triglyceride levels in diabetic rats.

White button mushrooms may also boost your immune system by enhancing the activity of natural killer cells, which attack viruses and tumors. In a study of Chinese women, those who ate at least 10 grams a day of fresh mushrooms — about one button mushroom — slashed their risk of breast cancer by 64 percent.

An Arizona State University lab study determined that ergothioneine, an antioxidant found in mushrooms, can protect against heart disease by interfering with processes that lead to the formation of fatty deposits in your arteries.

Begin the day with breakfast. Give yourself an energy boost by not skipping this important meal. But choose your breakfast foods wisely. Avoid sugary cereals or white toast and opt for oatmeal and other whole grains instead.

A recent Purdue University study suggests that including low-GI foods with breakfast helps prevent blood sugar spikes. In the study, people who ate a breakfast that included whole almonds felt fuller longer and had lower blood glucose concentrations after breakfast and lunch than those who did not eat a low-GI breakfast.

Don't stop with breakfast. To prevent dips in blood sugar throughout the day, try eating some quality carbs every four to five hours. This gives your body a constant source of fuel.

Curb caffeinated coffee. One part of breakfast you may want to rethink is coffee, or at least caffeinated coffee. One Canadian study of healthy young men found that caffeinated coffee impairs glucose tolerance, which means your blood sugar levels stay higher than normal. The effect is even greater when you drink it after a high-fat, high-calorie meal.

An earlier study by some of the same researchers found that drinking caffeinated coffee an hour before breakfast — whether breakfast consisted of a high-GI or low-GI cereal — negatively affected the body's blood sugar response compared to decaffeinated coffee.

Keep in mind that these studies involved only healthy young men, so the results may not apply to older people with diabetes. But it may not hurt to switch to decaf just in case.

Change your life for just $2 more a day

Tired of cutting out carbohydrates or trimming all the fat from your diet? Try eating more like someone from Greece, Italy, or the south of France. This pattern of eating, called the Mediterranean diet, is diverse and flavorful, featuring real food you love to eat — and real results you can see in weeks. Find out how this diet can help prevent or control diabetes and battle a wide range of other conditions.

Delve into the perfect diet. Unlike other eating plans, the Mediterranean diet doesn't have hard and fast rules. That's because the Greeks, French, and Italians don't eat exactly the same diet. But there are some helpful guidelines.

People who follow a Mediterranean diet usually get over 30 percent of their calories from fat — but the focus is on healthy monounsaturated fat, mostly from olive oil. You can also fill up on fruits, vegetables, fish, whole grains, beans, nuts, seeds, yogurt and other low-fat dairy products, and flavorful herbs and spices, while eating red meat and sweets only sparingly. Regular physical activity and moderate wine consumption — two glasses a day for a man or one for a woman — also contribute to the Mediterranean lifestyle.

This healthy lifestyle can cost a bit more. A Spanish study determined that eating the Mediterranean way costs more than eating a typical Western diet. For every 1,000 calories, expect to pay 90 cents more in daily food costs. Assuming a 2,000-calorie diet, that adds up to $1.80, or about $2, a day.

While you may pay more now, chances are you'll save money in the long run. That's because sticking to a Mediterranean diet can keep you healthy so you don't have to spend as much on doctors and medication. It's an easy way to spend just $2 more a day on groceries, and save thousands in medical bills.

Dodge diabetes. Any diet that helps you lose weight will also help fight diabetes. But a Mediterranean eating plan may be especially helpful in preventing and controlling diabetes.

Your chances of developing diabetes and heart disease increase if you have a group of risk factors known as metabolic syndrome. If you have any three of the following, you have metabolic syndrome.

- blood pressure of 130/85 or higher

- fasting blood sugar of 100 or higher

- waist circumference of at least 35 inches for women or 40 inches for men

- HDL, or good cholesterol, below 50 for women or below 40 for men

- triglycerides of 150 or higher

A recent Greek study of more than 2,000 people found that following a Mediterranean diet reduced the risk of metabolic syndrome by 20 percent. Interestingly, people with diabetes or heart disease were less likely to follow a Mediterranean diet.

Researchers who analyzed 50 previous studies also found that a Mediterranean diet helps lower the risk of metabolic syndrome. It also has positive effects on metabolic syndrome's individual components, including abdominal obesity, HDL and triglyceride levels, blood pressure, and blood sugar. The antioxidant and anti-inflammatory effects of the Mediterranean diet as a whole — as well as the beneficial effects of specific foods like olive oil, fruits, vegetables, fish, and whole grains — could get the credit.

Even if you already have diabetes, a Mediterranean diet can help. In an Italian study of 215 overweight people who had recently been diagnosed with type 2 diabetes, those who ate a Mediterranean-style diet were less likely to need blood sugar-lowering drugs than those who ate a low-fat diet. The monounsaturated fat from olive oil may improve insulin sensitivity, delaying the need for drug therapy. People on the Mediterranean diet also lost more weight and had greater improvements in blood sugar control and heart disease risk factors.

Stifle inflammation. Diabetes isn't the only condition that a Mediterranean diet helps fight. Arthritis, heart attack, cancer, and digestive problems are just some of the others. All of these diseases and more have a single contributing factor — inflammation. Read the newest research findings about how to stop this sneaky killer now.

Inflammation helps your body's immune system fight infection or injury. But chronic inflammation puts your health in peril. In addition to metabolic syndrome and diabetes, chronic inflammation has been linked to heart disease, cancer, arthritis, physical disability, and Alzheimer's disease.

Losing weight represents your best defense against inflammation, but some foods may help, too. And many of those foods — including olive oil, fish, nuts, legumes, fruits, vegetables, and whole grains — are found in the Mediterranean diet.

A recent Australian review pointed out that populations that consume a Mediterranean diet have lower incidences of chronic inflammatory diseases. Olive oil, thanks to its many phenolic compounds, plays a key role in protecting your health. One particular compound in olive oil called oleocanthal has similar anti-inflammatory properties as ibuprofen.

Long-term consumption of olive oil as part of a Mediterranean eating plan may help reduce the risk of chronic inflammation and its related conditions.

Look at the label. Olive oil is an amazing health food, but not all brands are created equal. Start by looking for the phrase "extra virgin" and eyeing the harvest date on the label to be sure you're getting all the health benefits you expect.

- Extra virgin oil is what emerges the first time the olives are pressed without using chemicals or high heat. It packs more antioxidants than other grades of olive oil.

- The harvest date indicates freshness. The older the oil, the fewer nutrients it contains. Look for a bottle dated the same year you're buying it. No harvest date? Choose a bottle with a "best by" date furthest away.

Sidestep olive oil imposters

Even when you think you know which olive oil you're buying, you may be in for a surprise. Labels can be misleading. Researchers at the University of California, Davis tested 19 different brands of olive oil, with surprising results. All claimed to be extra virgin, but eight out of 10 were not. Most imported oils failed the test. Nine out of 10 California olive oils passed.

You might be surprised at which brands made the cut. Sam's Club Kirkland Organic brand as well as Walmart's Great Value 100% both passed. So did Corto, California Olive Ranch, McEvoy Ranch Organic, and Lucero (Ascolano). Some of the biggest, best-known brands on grocery shelves failed. Some failed because they had been cut with cheaper, lower-grade oil. Others failed because they had begun to break down from age, exposure to light or heat, or improper storage.

Tom Mueller, olive oil connoisseur and author of the book *Extra Virginity: The sublime and scandalous world of olive oil* offers these tips for getting the freshest, most nutritious product.

- Only buy olive oil that comes in a dark, opaque bottle. Light passing through a clear bottle will break down the oil faster.

- Find an olive mill near you and buy your oil directly from there. California, Texas, Oregon, Georgia, Arizona, and Florida all boast active ones.

- Look for brands with Protected Designation of Origin (PDO; DOP in Italian) certification, or with Protected Geographical Indication (PGI; IGP in Italian) certification. These oils undergo strict quality control and are more likely to be real extra virgin. Oils certified by national or state olive oil associations, such as the California Olive Oil Council, are also good bets.

Make smart swaps. Here are five simple shopping-list substitutions that can turn your health around, fast. Fight weight gain, diabetes, heart disease, and much more by swapping Western-style diet staples for Mediterranean diet alternatives. Next time you're at the grocery store, choose:

- olive oil instead of margarine or butter.

- fish instead of red meat.

- whole grains, like brown rice, instead of refined grains, like white rice.

- low-fat dairy products, including yogurt, cheese, and milk, instead of full-fat versions.

- nuts and legumes instead of meat.

Popular grain boosts diabetes risk

Eat too much white rice, and you may be waving the white flag of surrender in the battle against diabetes.

A recent Harvard study suggests that higher white rice consumption leads to a higher risk of type 2 diabetes. Researchers examined four previous studies from China, Japan, Australia, and the United States. The link seemed stronger for Asians, probably because they eat much more rice. For the overall population, each serving of white rice a day increased the risk of diabetes by 11 percent.

White rice could boost your diabetes risk because of its high glycemic index (GI) value, which measures how quickly a food raises your blood sugar. White rice also has less fiber, magnesium, and vitamins than minimally processed whole grains like brown rice. Fiber and magnesium have been linked to a lower risk of diabetes.

You don't have to give up white rice completely, but consider swapping it for brown rice and other whole grains whenever possible.

Surprising ways to save your kidneys

People with diabetes find themselves at greater risk for kidney disease. But even if you don't have diabetes, you may be damaging your kidneys without even realizing it. Here's how to keep your kidneys running in tiptop condition. Following these tips helps prevent kidney stones — and more.

Stymie blood sugar. High blood sugar can damage your kidneys. In fact, diabetes is the leading cause of kidney failure in the United States.

When your blood sugar levels are high, more blood goes to your kidneys and forces them to work harder than usual. High blood sugar also damages blood vessels within the kidneys. Your overtaxed kidneys slowly lose their ability to filter waste and clean poisons from your blood.

One of the first signs of kidney disease is excess protein in the urine. A simple urine test can help detect that. Fortunately, if you get your high blood sugar under control early, your kidneys can return to functioning normally. But if your blood sugar stays high for several years, your kidneys could be permanently harmed.

Aim for a blood sugar target of 7 percent or below on the hemoglobin A1c test, or HbA1c, to prevent kidney disease or slow its progression. Diet, exercise, and medications can help you achieve this goal.

Bring down blood pressure. Like high blood sugar, high blood pressure takes its toll on your kidneys. Diabetes and high blood pressure rank as the two main risk factors for kidney disease. By damaging the blood vessels in your kidneys' filters, high blood pressure weakens your kidney function. This, in turn, often causes your blood pressure to go up even more, which further damages your kidneys.

Strive for a blood pressure reading of less than 130/80 — lower than the official high blood pressure cutoff of 140/90 — to prevent kidney disease or slow loss of kidney function. One way to help lower blood pressure without drugs is to restrict your salt intake. Limit sodium to 1,500 milligrams (mg) a day.

Pop fewer pain pills. Taking pain relievers soothes your pain now, but it may also lead to kidney problems later. Nonsteroidal anti-inflammatory drugs (NSAIDs), such as ibuprofen and naproxen, have been linked to kidney damage.

Recently, a Harvard study found that long-term use of these NSAIDs may increase the risk of kidney cancer. Overall, regular use of NSAIDs meant a 51-percent greater risk of developing kidney cancer during the 16-year study.

The longer you rely on these drugs, the higher your risk. For example, people who took NSAIDs daily for less than four years actually had a 19-percent lower risk of kidney cancer. But if they took them every day for between four and 10 years, their risk jumped to 36 percent greater. And people who used these pain relievers daily for 10 years or more nearly tripled their risk. Acetaminophen and the NSAID aspirin did not pose a similar threat.

Keep in mind that the overall risk for kidney cancer is small, with smoking and obesity the biggest risk factors. But you still may want to take some precautions, especially if you rely on NSAIDs daily. To protect yourself, try switching to acetaminophen. Or take the lowest effective dose of your usual NSAID — but have your doctor monitor your kidney function if you take them for long periods of time.

Drink less diet soda. It may seem like a smart move to cut calories and slash sugar by sipping diet soft drinks. But drinking two or more servings a day of artificially sweetened soda may double your risk for poor kidney function.

That's what a Harvard Medical School study of 3,256 women participating in the Nurses' Health Study found. In the study, a serving could be a glass, a can, or a bottle of a beverage. Luckily, drinking less than two diet sodas a day did not seem to put your kidneys in danger.

Refreshing drink comes with risk

There's nothing like a cold glass of iced tea to cool down on a hot summer day. But you may want to rethink your beverage of choice — especially if you're prone to forming kidney stones.

A recent Loyola University study pointed out that iced tea contains high concentrations of oxalate, a chemical that contributes to the formation of kidney stones. While drinking fluids helps prevent kidney stones, drinking too much iced tea may actually make things worse. Hot tea also contains oxalates, but most people don't drink enough of it to cause kidney stones.

That doesn't mean you have to avoid iced tea entirely. An occasional glass of iced tea is probably fine, but don't overdo it. Drink plenty of water to stay hydrated instead.

Use caution with calcium. You may take calcium supplements to ward off osteoporosis. But while you're protecting your bones, you may be making yourself more vulnerable to painful kidney stones. Studies suggest that getting too much calcium from supplements increases your risk of developing kidney stones. However, calcium from foods may help lower your risk.

In one study, women who received 1,000 milligrams (mg) of supplementary calcium each day for seven years — on top of any calcium they got from their diet — were 17 percent more likely to develop kidney stones than women who did not supplement their diets with calcium. But women in the study who got the most calcium from foods slashed their risk of kidney stones by 65 percent compared to those who ate the least. The participants in the study who took calcium supplements also took 400 IU (international units) of vitamin D every day.

A University of Washington study of older women also found that dietary calcium had a protective effect. Women who ate the most calcium at the start of the study were 28 percent less likely to develop kidney stones compared to those whose diets contained the least.

Good food sources of calcium include milk, yogurt, and cheese. You can also find it in calcium-fortified foods, such as orange juice and cereal. Drinking more fluids and cutting down on salt are also helpful strategies for preventing kidney stones.

If you need to take calcium supplements, take them with meals to minimize the risk of developing kidney stones. Often, women who take supplementary calcium also take vitamin D, which helps your body absorb calcium. But high blood levels of vitamin D may also boost your risk of developing kidney stones. Talk to your doctor before starting or stopping any supplement regimen.

Minimize risk of medical procedures. Tests and screenings help doctors detect disease, but sometimes those tests end up causing trouble for your kidneys.

Certain medical imaging exams use contrast agents, or dyes, such as barium or iodine, that can cause temporary kidney damage. However, a recent study suggests that these contrast agents may have longer-lasting consequences — including heart attack, stroke, or end-stage kidney disease.

Some oral sodium phosphate products used to clear your bowels before a colonoscopy have been linked to a rare but serious form of kidney failure. Ask your doctor about safer phosphate-free alternatives.

Steer clear of unexpected source of lead

Thanks to federal regulations, you may not have to worry about lead in gasoline, canned foods, paint, or pipes anymore. But if you enjoy shopping in antique or vintage stores, you may get an unwelcome blast from the past. That's because old jewelry, toys, kitchenware, and knickknacks may be hiding unhealthy amounts of lead.

In a recent study, researchers purchased 28 used consumer items and analyzed them for lead content. They found that 19 of them exceeded the federal standards for lead. Alarmingly, items like these could contain more than 700 times the amount of lead currently allowed by law.

Lead exposure can lead to kidney damage, speeding the deterioration of your kidneys' ability to filter toxins from your blood. The effect is 15 times worse for people with type 2 diabetes.

Protect yourself by conducting a lead swab test on used items with kits available in hardware or home improvement stores.

---

7 unusual ways to fight diabetes

Eating a healthy diet, exercising regularly, and maintaining a healthy weight still rank as tried-and-true methods to prevent diabetes. But for even more protection, try these unusual tricks to lower your risk.

Stop sitting so much. Stand up to diabetes by standing up more often. A recent British study found that women who stay seated for long periods of time every day are more prone to developing diabetes. They had higher levels of insulin, C-reactive protein, and other signs of inflammation that act as precursors to developing diabetes. Even when time spent exercising was taken into account, the link between excessive sitting and diabetes warning signs remained.

Luckily, you can improve your fitness by fidgeting and other types of "incidental physical activity," according to a Canadian study. Movements that are not formally exercise — such as pulling weeds, chopping vegetables, bobbing your foot while you sit, and pacing — can contribute to better fitness. Find ways to fit more movement into your day. Consider parking further away or taking the stairs rather than the elevator.

Beware of BPA. Bisphenol A (BPA), a chemical found in some hard plastic containers and the linings of metal cans, may boost your risk of diabetes. A West Virginia study found that those with the highest levels of BPA in their urine had a 50-percent greater risk of developing diabetes compared to those with the lowest.

In another study, one 12-ounce serving of canned soup per day for five straight days boosted urinary BPA levels by more than 1,000 percent.

Cutting back on eating canned foods is the best way to limit BPA exposure. But BPA is also found in a surprising variety of paper products — including napkins, toilet paper, lottery tickets, food wrappers, newspapers, magazines, boarding passes, and especially receipts. Wash your hands after handling a receipt, and wear gloves if you're a cashier.

Bulk up. Don't just lose fat. Build more muscle. That's the message from a UCLA study that found that muscle mass is key to lowering your diabetes risk. Researchers found that for each 10-percent increase in the ratio of muscle mass to total body weight, insulin resistance went down by 11 percent and pre-diabetes symptoms by 12 percent.

Embrace extra-virgin. Fried food is rarely healthy, but food fried in extra-virgin olive oil may help improve your post-meal insulin response.

In an Italian study, 12 obese, insulin-resistant women and five lean women ate two different meals. Both included pasta, zucchini, apples, and olive oil. But one featured grilled zucchini and uncooked oil, while the other meal used the same amount of oil to stir-fry the pasta and deep-fry the zucchini. The two meals did not affect the lean women differently, but the fried meal led to a reduced insulin response among obese women.

Sidestep statins. Statins lower your cholesterol, but they may also boost your risk of developing diabetes. In a recent study of 153,840 women ages 50 to 79 participating in the Women's Health Initiative, statin use was linked to a 48-percent greater risk of diabetes.

Make sure you try to control your cholesterol through lifestyle changes, such as diet and exercise, before resorting to statins. Your doctor should weigh the risks and benefits of statins before prescribing them.

Forget fragrance. Products that contain "fragrance" may smell good — but they stink when it comes to diabetes. That's because they contain phthalates. These chemicals are found in a variety of products, including cosmetics, shampoos, soaps, lubricants, pesticides, paints, plastics, toys, packaging, raincoats, shower curtains, and scented candles. They may even find their way into your food from plastic wrappers.

That's bad news because studies suggest a link between phthalate exposure and diabetes. In one study of American men, those with abdominal obesity and insulin resistance — two forerunners of diabetes — were more likely to have higher concentrations of phthalate substances in their urine.

A recent Swedish study of more than 1,000 70-year-old men and women found that those with higher blood phthalate levels had roughly twice the risk of developing diabetes as those with lower levels.

It's hard to avoid phthalates entirely, but you can limit your exposure by avoiding products that contain fragrance or dibutyl phthalate (DBP). Use a non-vinyl shower curtain, paint in well-ventilated areas, and don't cook or microwave your food in plastic.

Spend more time in the sun. Boosting your vitamin D levels may boost your defense against diabetes. A German study found that people with the highest blood levels of vitamin D slashed their risk of developing diabetes by 37 percent compared to those with the lowest. Vitamin D may help by squelching the inflammation that contributes to diabetes.

Your body produces vitamin D when you get enough exposure to sunlight, so spending more time in the sun can help. So can taking supplements. You can also find vitamin D in foods like oily fish, eggs, and fortified dairy products.

Set aside the saltshaker. Restricting salt helps prevent high blood pressure and stroke, but it may also help lower your diabetes risk. That's because a high-salt diet promotes insulin resistance.

One good way to cut down on salt is to give up processed meats. These include hot dogs, bacon, sausage, deli meats, pepperoni, and any meat smoked, salted, cured, or chemically preserved. A Finnish study found that eating processed meat raised diabetes risk by 37 percent over a 12-year period. Researchers suspect the sodium content of the processed meat was to blame.

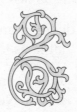

Digestive disorders: terrific tummy tamers

Soothe surprising causes of stomach pain

You've tried everything, but the bloating, diarrhea, or abdominal pain won't go away. And no doctor can seem to find the cause. If this sounds familiar, then a common medication or little-known food sensitivity could be to blame. Fortunately, a few tweaks could soothe your symptoms.

Monitor heartburn medicines. People taking proton pump inhibitors (PPIs), typically for heartburn, ulcers, and gastro-esophageal reflux disease (GERD), may be more likely to develop *Clostridium difficile*. This type of infection causes diarrhea, abdominal pain, and fever.

Experts aren't sure why, but PPIs including omeprazole (Prilosec), esomeprazole (Nexium), rabeprazole (AcipHex), lansoprazole (Prevacid), and pantoprazole (Protonix), among others, seem to raise your risk of catching it. Play it safe with these precautions.

- Take the lowest dose of PPI that will control your symptoms.

- Take it only for as long as needed to treat your condition.

- See a doctor if you develop any *C. difficile* symptoms, including diarrhea that lasts longer than three days.

Balance out acidic foods. Cut back on high-acid foods, and you might not need heartburn drugs. New evidence suggests they could bear the blame for some types of reflux — specifically laryngopharyngeal reflux.

Unlike GERD, laryngopharyngeal reflux usually happens during the day, not at night, and it doesn't always cause a burning sensation. Instead, it leads to hoarseness, a sore throat, and chronic coughing.

A small study tested a low-acid diet in 20 people with this form of reflux who weren't helped by traditional drugs, such as PPIs and H2 blockers. Loading up on low-acid foods and limiting high-acid ones improved symptoms in 19 out of 20 people. Three saw their symptoms completely disappear. The diet was strict. For two weeks, people:

- ate only low-acid foods, like skim milk, turkey breast, rice, potatoes, oatmeal, honey, chicken, fish, celery, beans, and whole grain or rye breads.

- were allowed to drink only one cup of coffee a day.

- could not eat any fruits other than melons and bananas.

- completely avoided red meat, butter, cheese, fried foods, high-fat meat, carbonated soda, citrus fruit, and hot pepper sauces.

Experts say after following this plan for two to four weeks, you can slowly add back some fattier foods that would normally aggravate reflux, such as cheese, eggs, meats, or sauces. But make sure your overall meals stay focused on low-acid foods. When you do eat acidic foods, like strawberries, be sure to pair them with nonacidic foods like cereal and low-fat milk. Skip anything that comes out of bottles or cans whenever possible. Almost all of these are acidic, thanks to the preservatives added to them.

Suspect a gluten sensitivity. Experts now know you can be sensitive to gluten, the main protein in wheat, rye, and barley, without having celiac disease. In both conditions, eating gluten triggers an immune system reaction. Unlike celiac, gluten sensitivity doesn't usually damage your small intestine.

You're likely to suffer with diarrhea and abdominal pain after indulging in gluten-filled foods, but these other symptoms may surprise you.

- changes in behavior
- bone or joint pain
- muscle cramps
- chronic fatigue
- weight loss
- depression
- anemia
- skin rash
- brain fog
- headaches
- numbness in your fingers, arms, or legs

Get tested for celiac disease first to rule it out. It shares some of the same symptoms. Next, try cutting all gluten-containing foods from your diet. Then slowly add them back a little at a time, and see if your symptoms return. If so, you'll know you are sensitive to gluten.

Find your Fodmap tolerance. A new plan known as the low-Fodmap diet could be the next big breakthrough in irritable bowel syndrome (IBS) treatment. Fodmap stands

How to spot gluten in cosmetics

Makeup or lotion made with gluten could cause a rash, bloating, or diarrhea in people with celiac disease. The danger lies mostly with hand lotions and lipsticks that could get into your mouth, or with skin lesions that could absorb gluten into your body.

Some experts are skeptical that cosmetics could pose a problem, but if you're concerned, try these tips.

- Check the ingredients list for the words "wheat," "barley," "malt," "rye," "oat," "triticum vulgare," "hordeum vulgare," "secale cereale," and "avena sativa."

- No list on the container? Look for a product information sheet near the display, or call the manufacturer and ask if the product contains anything made from oats, wheat, rye, or barley.

- Buy cosmetics and lotions specifically labeled gluten-free.

for "fermentable oligosaccharides, disaccharides, monosaccharides, and polyols." These sugars can cause problems for three reasons.

- Your gut has trouble absorbing them.

- Bacteria ferment them, producing gas, bloating, and abdominal pain.

- They draw more water into your intestines, which can lead to diarrhea.

Cutting Fodmaps from your diet can reduce gas in just one or two days, since gas is caused by fermentation in the gut. That reduces bloating, the main cause of abdominal pain in IBS. This special diet also brings the bacteria in your intestines back into healthy balance, a known problem for people with IBS.

You begin by avoiding all foods high in Fodmaps for four to six weeks. Then you add them back slowly until you find which sugars aggravate your IBS. A British study showed that following a low-Fodmap diet improved people's IBS symptoms more than the standard advice, such as cutting back on caffeine, alcohol, dairy, resistant starches, fatty foods, fizzy drinks, and sorbitol, or increasing your fiber intake.

A whopping 86 percent of IBS sufferers saw their symptoms improve on the low-Fodmap diet, with less bloating, abdominal pain, and gas than those on the standard diet. Half of the standard group either saw no improvement or had their symptoms worsen.

To find out if it could help you, start by getting a breath test. This measures the gas produced in your intestines. It can tell you which, if any, sugars you have problems with. Once you know your triggers, you can avoid them. This table of foods highest in Fodmaps can help you get started.

Fodmap	Top food sources
fructans (fructo-oligosaccharides)	wheat, rye, onions, garlic, artichokes
galacto-oligosaccharides	legumes
lactose	milk
fructose	honey, apples, pears, watermelon, mango
sorbitol	apples, pears, stone fruits, sugar-free gum and mints
mannitol	mushrooms, cauliflower, sugar-free gum and mints

The next step is to find a dietician trained in the low-Fodmap eating plan. They can help you spot Fodmaps in fresh and packaged foods as well as medications. Medical centers at some colleges and universities offer Fodmap help, too. Or get advice from other IBS sufferers through an online support group such as *www.ibsgroup.org*.

Avoid alcohol. Even moderate amounts of alcohol — one drink a day for women, two for men — may lead to an overgrowth of bacteria in your small intestines, a condition known as small intestinal bacterial overgrowth (SIBO). It's marked by bloating, gas, abdominal pain, constipation, and diarrhea. SIBO can even cause nutritional deficiencies, as the bacteria gobble up nutrients your body needs for itself.

The link between moderate drinking and SIBO isn't certain. More research is needed. Experts also don't know if avoiding alcohol will improve SIBO symptoms. A course of antibiotics or probiotics might, though, so talk to your doctor about getting relief.

New hope for hard-to-treat bowel problems

Inflammatory bowel disease (IBD) is no fun. Once you have it, it can't be cured. It can, however, be tamed and treated. New research points to natural ways of preventing IBD, treating the symptoms, and limiting the damage it does in your gut.

IBD is different from irritable bowel syndrome (IBS). It's an autoimmune disorder that causes inflammation along your digestive tract. The two share some symptoms, but unlike IBS, IBD can actually damage the intestines.

Doctors suspect it's caused by a combination of genetics and the things around you. Certain genes make you prone to developing IBD. Then one day, something in your environment, perhaps a food allergy or an infection, triggers your immune system to attack your digestive tract — only the system never turns off properly. It keeps attacking.

IBD takes many forms. The two most common are Crohn's disease and ulcerative colitis.

- Crohn's causes inflammation in the upper half of the digestive tract, mostly in the small intestine.

- Ulcerative colitis affects the lower half, inflaming the large intestine, including the colon and rectum.

Both are marked by abdominal pain and bloody diarrhea, though colitis can also cause nausea, vomiting, and fever. And both can lead to far more serious complications, including ulcers and perforated bowels. Luckily, there's good news. New research suggests certain foods and supplements may help curb flare-ups and even prevent IBD in the first place.

Is it IBS or something else?

It's easy to confuse the symptoms of irritable bowel syndrome (IBS) with other problems, especially after age 50. Make sure you get the right diagnosis. Instead of IBS, you may have:

- colon polyps, colon cancer, or ulcerative colitis. A colonoscopy or sigmoidoscopy can determine this.

- celiac disease, if your symptoms mostly involve diarrhea or alternating diarrhea and constipation. A blood test can diagnose celiac.

- lactose intolerance, if your symptoms seem to worsen after eating dairy or packaged foods made with it. A breath test can confirm lactose intolerance.

The opposite can also happen. You may get diagnosed with one of these conditions, when in reality you have IBS. Diverticulitis, Crohn's disease, intestinal obstruction, and infections of the digestive tract can also be mistaken for IBS.

Clear up Crohn's with CLA. Conjugated linoleic acid is naturally found in meat and dairy foods, but a small study shows that CLA supplements could help treat Crohn's disease.

Thirteen people with mild to moderate Crohn's took a 6-gram (g) dose of CLA every day for three months, in addition to their normal IBD medications. Half said their symptoms and quality of life noticeably improved. Best of all, CLA seemed to help without causing side effects.

This compound cools inflammation and quiets the backfiring immune system signals behind IBD. After 12 weeks, CLA supplements had helped stop immune cells from pumping out inflammatory compounds.

The supplements used in this study contained two types of CLA — cis-9, trans-11 isomers and cis-12, trans-10 isomers. Check labels to make sure yours does, too. Supplements made from safflower oil tend to have the same half-and-half mix.

CLA may worsen blood sugar control if you are obese or have diabetes, so take it under a doctor's supervision.

Soak up the sunshine vitamin. Women who lived in the northern United States at age 30 were more likely to develop IBD than those living in the South, according to a new study. Southern-dwellers were half as likely to get Crohn's disease and one-third as likely to get ulcerative colitis. Sunshine boosts vitamin D in your blood, which could explain this IBD Mason-Dixon line.

- This nutrient is key to healthy immune system responses. It helps regulate T cells, the immune cells that churn out inflammatory compounds in IBD.

- It also helps maintain the inner lining that protects your intestines. That could be crucial to preventing IBD.

The vitamin D connection may also explain why people with IBD experience seasonal flare-ups. Ulcerative colitis tends to be at its worst in December, while Crohn's causes more trouble in autumn and winter, when the sunny days of summer begin to shorten.

Of course, a shortage of vitamin D in your body could be a symptom of IBD, not the cause. People with IBD often have trouble absorbing vitamin D from food. And if you're not feeling well, you are less likely to get outside in the sunlight.

Still, it's worth discussing this link with your doctor if you suffer from Crohn's or colitis. She can test your blood levels of vitamin D and suggest a supplement, if needed. A small study found that taking 10,000 international units (IU) of vitamin D daily for six months improved Crohn's symptoms in people who were deficient. Have your doctor monitor your intake, as this nutrient can be toxic in large amounts.

Eat apples — peel and all. Polyphenols, natural compounds in apple peels, may protect against colitis. Mice were given a drug known to cause ulcerative colitis, but those fed apple polyphenols never developed the disease. These compounds seemed to block the inflammation that triggers IBD, and suppress T cells in the colon, helping protect this part of the large intestine.

"It appears that the old adage rings true in more ways than one," says John Wherry, deputy editor of the *Journal of Leukocyte Biology*, which published this research. "In addition to the obvious health benefits of the nutrients and fiber in fruits and vegetables, this study indicates that even something as relatively common as the apple contains other healthy ingredients that can have serious therapeutic value."

Bring on the broccoli. Cruciferous vegetables such as broccoli and Brussels sprouts may guard your gut against immune disorders like IBD. Special cells line your intestines, defending it against infections and repairing any damage. Having too little of a substance called AhR causes a sharp drop in the number of these protective cells. That's where food comes in. How many vegetables you eat may directly affect how much AhR you have.

"After feeding otherwise healthy mice a vegetable-poor diet for two to three weeks, I was amazed to see 70 to 80 percent of these protective cells disappear," says Marc Veldhoen, an immunologist at The Babraham Institute in Cambridge, England.

Losing these cells upsets the balance of bacteria in your digestive system and leaves your gut lining vulnerable to damage. Fortunately, eating cruciferous vegetables naturally raises your AhR levels.

Make friends with fiber. Getting more soluble fiber in your daily diet can also bring balance to your gut bacteria. That, in turn, could help prevent diseases like IBD.

Researchers had 20 healthy men either boost their intake of fiber to 35 grams (g) a day, or stay at their normal amount of 14 g. To up their intake, the men ate snack bars containing 21 g of soluble fiber daily. Eating high-fiber snack bars led to the growth of more health-promoting bacteria.

"For example, one type of bacteria that thrived as a result of the types of fiber fed in this study is inherently anti-inflammatory," says Kelly Swanson, professor of animal science at the University of Illinois. Snack bars made with soluble corn fiber were especially beneficial.

Fiber doesn't get absorbed into the bloodstream like other nutrients. It travels to your gut, where bacteria feast on it and ferment it, pumping out healthy compounds. Researchers say the bacteria that thrived on fiber in this study are the same types found in a healthy digestive tract.

The bacteria living in your gut can make you more or less susceptible to illnesses such as IBD and colon cancer, as well as nondigestive conditions like type 2 diabetes and rheumatoid arthritis. "When we understand what kinds of fiber best nurture these health-promoting bacteria, we should be able to modify imbalances to support and improve gastrointestinal health," explains Swanson.

"Unfortunately, people eat only about half of the 30 to 35 grams of daily fiber that is recommended," he says. "To achieve these health benefits, consumers should read nutrition labels and choose foods that have high fiber content."

Check with your doctor first if high-fiber foods like raw fruits and vegetables aggravate your IBD symptoms.

Heart disease: tactics to keep your ticker in top shape

6 kitchen gadgets that can save your heart

You want to cook heart-healthy meals, but you worry about how much extra time and energy that will take. Relax. Timesaving kitchen gadgets can make those meals a snap to prepare and delicious to eat. To help you decide which gadgets are worth buying, consider these no-nonsense choices, and learn how to combine them with the right foods to help prevent heart attacks and strokes.

Whip up blueberry smoothies with a blender. You probably know that veggies, like raw carrots and broccoli, are full of cancer-fighting, heart-healing nutrients called antioxidants. But do you know that wild blueberries are packed with as much antioxidant power as five servings of those vegetables? That makes blueberries one of nature's best sources of antioxidants. But that's not the only reason you'll want them in your smoothie.

Eating just one cup of blueberries every week can reduce your risk of developing high blood pressure. Blueberries also help prevent the oxidation of LDL cholesterol, a key step in developing hardening of the arteries. Together with their ability to help lower cholesterol, these powers make blueberries an excellent anti-stroke and anti-heart-disease food. They may also help prevent diabetes and colon cancer.

To take advantage of these health-defending powers, make a delicious breakfast smoothie with a half cup each of blueberries, nonfat vanilla yogurt, milk or orange juice, and ice or a frozen banana. Your blender can make all kinds of smoothies, including mixed fruit smoothies with hidden vegetables. Use it for salad dressings, healthy sandwich spreads, hummus, and soups like gazpacho as well.

Make overnight oatmeal in the slow cooker. If nature's most perfect foods are the ones that help you live longer, oatmeal may be one of the best. A recent study suggests people who eat a lot of oatmeal may have a lower risk of dying. Oatmeal's fiber may be the reason why. The study found that people who ate the most fiber had the least risk of dying from heart disease, lung disease, infections, or any other cause over a nine-year period.

To add more fiber to your diet, do it the easy way. At bedtime, put one part steel-cut oats and four parts water in a small slow cooker, set the cooker on low, and let cook overnight. Add toppings like raisins, berries, or nuts the next morning.

Try overnight cooking for other fiber-rich cooked cereals like barley, buckwheat, or even brown rice. You can also use the slow cooker to cook chicken, turkey, lean cuts of beef, soups, stews, and chili. The American Heart Association even created a slow cooker cookbook to help.

Find deep discounts on pricey kitchen gadgets

You can find astonishing discounts on expensive kitchen gadgets if they're labeled as "refurbished" or "factory reconditioned," but do your homework first. Items with this label have been returned to the seller for reasons ranging from "duplicate gift" or "wrong color" to "does not work."

Look for refurbished products at outlet stores, the manufacturer's website, and Overstock.com. Before you snap up a refurbished item, find out its normal price range, and read product or user reviews. Avoid items with a reputation for poor quality or breakdowns.

Also, look for a full warranty that matches the new product warranty and a return policy with a full refund and reasonable return period. Make sure all accessories and manuals are included in the original box. Inspect and test the product if possible, or check whether it has been quality-inspected after refurbishing.

Steam vegetables with the microwave. Never eat mushy vegetables again. Steam them instead for a farm-fresh taste and texture. Start with broccoli, the amazing vegetable you can get anywhere. It does everything from helping your heart pump better and helping prevent cancer to boosting your immune system.

Broccoli even helps head off blood vessel damage in people with diabetes. This damage occurs because high blood sugar helps cell-damaging free radical molecules multiply inside your blood vessels. But a British study found that the sulforaphane in broccoli helps protect blood vessels from free radicals. If you have diabetes, this may defend your blood vessels against damage and help protect you from heart attacks and strokes.

To steam broccoli, put chopped broccoli or florets plus two tablespoons of water into a microwave-safe dish. Cover and place in the microwave. Cook on high for three minutes and check for doneness. The time needed for steaming depends on how powerful your microwave is, so you may need to cook it another minute or two. Keep checking until the broccoli is cooked to your satisfaction.

This method works for other healthy vegetables, too. Try it and discover just how good vegetables can be. If you don't have a microwave, consider buying an inexpensive countertop steamer with single- or double-decker steaming baskets, or spend even less and buy a steamer basket that fits inside large pots.

Enjoy fresh-squeezed OJ from the juicer. Orange juice from your home juicer delivers a vibrant taste and vitamin C without the extra sugars you sometimes get from juice drinks at the supermarket. That's good news because researchers found that people with the highest blood levels of vitamin C were half as likely to die during a four-year period as people with the lowest levels. Experts think adding just 1.75 ounces of vitamin C-rich produce to your diet each day could reduce your risk of death from any cause by 20 percent. But that's not all this vitamin can do for you.

- People with the highest blood levels of vitamin C slashed their stroke risk by 42 percent over 10 years, one study reported.

- Three recent studies suggest vitamin C may play a role in helping prevent prostate cancer, especially vitamin C from food.

- This vitamin can even keep your skin young. Women over 39 who took in the most vitamin C were less likely to have wrinkles and dry skin, a British study reported.

- Regularly taking in high amounts of vitamin C may help prevent infections, especially in older adults with low levels.

To add vitamin C to your diet, make juice from oranges, tangerines, and other citrus fruits. You can make a great lemonade by juicing half a lemon with three apples. But that's just the beginning. Make unusual juices such as beet juice, which may help high blood pressure. Combine sweet fruits with vegetables like carrots, celery, spinach, or cucumbers for an extra-nutritious juice treat.

You can also make juice sodas with seltzer water, or homemade versions of fruit punch, expensive green juices, or cherry juice. Add the leftover fruit or vegetable pulp to baked goods, pasta sauce, or stews, or toss it into your compost pile.

Cook black beans in the pressure cooker. Deliciously nutritious beans contain at least five vitamins and minerals including thiamin (vitamin B1), folate, iron, magnesium, and manganese. They are full of fiber, like soluble fiber that helps lower cholesterol. Bean fiber may also help bind toxins and help remove them from our bodies. A harvest of beans is even high in antioxidants. Antioxidants are a key factor in anti-aging because they help neutralize the free radicals that contribute to aging, hardening of the arteries, and heart disease.

Black beans have more antioxidants than most other beans, so give them a try. You may be tempted to buy canned black beans because they take less time to prepare, but canned beans contain sodium. Too much sodium can damage your blood vessels and raise your risk of high blood pressure.

So use dried black beans instead, and slash their cooking time by tossing them in a pressure cooker. Enjoy black beans in chili, Mexican dishes, soups, and stews, or mix them with rice and diced tomatoes. And don't forget other delicious bean dishes like red beans and rice, hummus, falafels, and baked beans.

Puree vegetables with an immersion blender. The American Heart Association recommends at least four-and-a-half cups of fresh fruit and vegetables daily. If you eat less than that, puree vegetables with an immersion blender, and slip the puree into soups, stews, pasta sauces, or casseroles for an extra daily serving.

The immersion blender or stick blender is a handheld wand with blender blades on one end. Use it to puree vegetables in a tall narrow bowl or glass, or even the pot you're cooking in. You can also use an immersion blender to make mashed potatoes, dips, pesto, hummus, pasta sauce, and soups like butternut squash or black bean.

Plan ahead and save

Small kitchen appliances usually go on sale during May or December. Keep an eye on your favorite products and their prices so you can be ready to pounce when that May clearance or December holiday sale arrives.

---

5 surprising things you should know about cholesterol

Scientists are finding out cholesterol doesn't always behave the way they expect. Low cholesterol is not always good, and high cholesterol is not always bad. What's more, some of the secrets for controlling cholesterol may surprise you. To help clear up the confusion, here are five unexpected things your doctor may not tell you about cholesterol.

High LDL increases dementia risk. You may already know that total cholesterol above 200 or "bad" LDL cholesterol above 129 raises your risk of heart attacks and strokes. But here's a surprise. High LDL cholesterol may also increase your risk of Alzheimer's disease and vascular dementia, which results from small strokes or severely narrowed arteries. Fortunately, raising your "good" HDL cholesterol can help. A recent study found that an HDL cholesterol of 56 or higher may lower your risk of Alzheimer's disease up to 60 percent.

Keeping HDL at 60 or higher not only lowers your risk of Alzheimer's disease, it reduces your risk of heart attack and stroke, too. Good ways to pump up HDL cholesterol include getting moderate exercise like brisk walking, losing weight if you are overweight, quitting smoking, and avoiding trans fats.

Cholesterol is linked to depression. Low cholesterol may raise your risk of two problems. Low HDL cholesterol below 40 for men or 50 for women may raise your risk of heart attacks and strokes. And a French study has found that low HDL cholesterol also raises the risk of depression in women age 65 and older.

The French study also revealed that men age 65 and older may double their risk of depression if their LDL — not HDL — cholesterol dips below 117, especially if they have a vulnerability in a serotonin transporter gene. This gene helps promote communication between brain cells, so your risk for depression rises if it is faulty. But don't change your LDL cholesterol goal based on this one study. Instead, talk to your doctor to learn more about your risk of depression, and find out the safest LDL cholesterol level for you.

You can flush fat from your arteries with tea. Drinking green tea lowers both total cholesterol and LDL cholesterol, according to recent research. Normally, your body reabsorbs cholesterol that reaches your intestines, but experts say the powerful catechin compounds in green tea allow the cholesterol to be swept out of your body. The catechins may even lower production of new cholesterol.

Green tea may also help you in another way. Cholesterol buildup on your artery walls can lead to hardened, narrowed blood vessels that cause heart attacks and strokes. Studies show how a daily glass of green tea can help prevent all that.

- High blood pressure can speed up narrowing and hardening of the arteries, but studies suggest a glass of green tea every day may help prevent you from developing high blood pressure.

- European research discovered that people who drank 8 ounces of tea a day were less likely to have severe narrowing of the arteries.

That means just one glass of green tea daily could be enough to keep your arteries smooth and supple. In fact, this one heart-smart drink can also lower high blood pressure and triglycerides, and help prevent the blood clots that trigger heart attacks and strokes. Enjoy green tea hot during the winter, and try it cold on steamy summer days.

There's something better than fish oil. One supplement out-performed fish oil in reducing cholesterol and triglycerides in recent animal studies. That supplement was krill oil, and the studies suggest it may produce bigger drops in cholesterol and triglycerides than fish oil can in the same amount of time. Krill oil comes from shrimp-like sea animals that make an oil rich in the omega-3 fats eicosapentaenoic acid (EPA) and docosahexaenoic acid (DHA). One type of krill, known as Antarctic krill, produces high levels of EPA and DHA. Because these fats come in a form called phospholipids, some studies and experts suggest your body may absorb and use them more readily.

Krill oil may have other benefits, too. Scientists have discovered that obese people have above-normal levels of the body's natural endocannabinoid compounds. Unfortunately, increased endocannabinoid levels have also been linked to appetite and eating larger amounts of food every day. But recent research found krill oil decreased one of these compounds in obese people. This suggests krill oil may have beneficial effects on endocannabinoid compounds, which also influence pain, mood, and memory.

Studies suggest 1 to 3 grams of krill oil daily may help reduce cholesterol. But talk to your doctor before you try this supplement. It may not be safe for people who take blood-thinning medications, like warfarin, and you should never take it if you are allergic to shellfish.

Apples and oranges help lower "bad" cholesterol. Feast on healthy fruit but don't throw away the part that is best for your heart. Some fruit skins may help lower "bad" LDL cholesterol because they contain a fiber called pectin. Pectin not only lowers LDL cholesterol, but total cholesterol, too. For best results, eat more apples and oranges, which have high pectin in their peels. This doesn't mean you have to eat orange peels. The pectin is in the white pith, not the orange-colored peel. When you remove the peel, leave as much of the pith as you can. If you prefer your pectin from apples, choose organic apples to make sure you avoid peels coated with wax or hidden pesticides — and don't forget to leave the peel on when you eat them.

Brew a perfect cup of green tea

If you make green tea the same way you make black tea, it will taste bitter. For better flavor, don't steep green tea in boiling water. Use water that is almost hot enough to boil, and only steep the tea for two to three minutes — not a moment longer. To add a different flavor to your green tea, add a splash of lemon or orange juice, a teaspoon of pure vanilla extract or honey, or mint leaves.

Exciting new ways to lower your blood pressure

High blood pressure shouldn't be a life sentence of bland, salt-free eating and boring workouts. Beating high blood pressure should include new foods and clever tricks to help push your blood pressure down. Even if you think you have already tried everything, these new ideas may surprise you.

Gain triple protection from grapes. You can lower your blood pressure and fight heart disease and diabetes just by eating delicious, refreshing Concord grapes or drinking their juice. A small Korean study found that men who drank Concord grape juice every day lowered their systolic blood pressure (the top number) 7.2 points and diastolic blood pressure (the bottom number) 6.2 points in eight weeks. But that's not all grapes can do.

Most people experience a natural dip in blood pressure during the night, but people who don't dip deeply enough have a higher risk of strokes and heart attacks. Fortunately, grape juice may help you reach a deep enough nightly low to improve your odds of good health and longevity.

In a Boston University study, people who drank grape juice experienced deeper nightly dips in blood pressure and a 2-point drop in blood sugar. For results like these, drink grape juice every day — about 6 ounces of Concord grape juice for every 55 pounds of body weight. That would be 12 ounces a day for a 110-pound woman or 24 ounces for a 220-pound man. Keep in mind a 6-ounce glass of grape juice has about 105 calories.

Turn your BP drug into a lifesaving medicine. Take your blood pressure medication at the wrong time of day, and it could be ineffective when you need it to save your life. According to a five-year study, people who took at least one of their blood-pressure-lowering medications at night reduced their risk of heart attack, stroke, or death from heart disease by 66 percent compared with people who took their medicines in the morning.

Taking medicine at night was particularly helpful to people who didn't experience a nightly dip in blood pressure. Those who took a blood pressure medicine at bedtime shifted closer to a normal nightly dip. In addition, taking medication at night helped keep blood pressure closer to normal during sleep. This is important because abnormal sleep-time blood pressure is a very good predictor of death from heart disease.

If you take all your blood-pressure-lowering medications in the morning, talk to your doctor about switching one of your drugs to bedtime. That change could save your life.

Help lower blood pressure with soda. Find a soda sweetened with stevia, and the sweetener may help you lower your blood pressure and blood sugar. Just be sure you know what to look for at the grocery store, or you may not get what you pay for.

Stevia is a "zero-calorie" sweetener made from the plant *Stevia rebaudiana*. Since 2008, the FDA has issued "Generally Recognized As Safe (GRAS) Letters of No Objection" for two stevia compounds, stevioside and rebaudioside A, allowing them to be used in soft drinks and other products. The "stevia" on a product's label may refer to either sweetener, but here is how the two compounds are very different.

Taking 250 milligram (mg) capsules of stevioside three times daily lowered systolic blood pressure 12 points and diastolic blood pressure 8 points, one study reported. A small study also suggests 1,000 mg of stevioside may significantly lower blood sugar. But 1,000 mg of rebaudiana-A had no effect on blood pressure or blood sugar in studies. So before you buy a soda sweetened with "stevia," check its ingredients on the label. If that doesn't reveal which stevia is inside, visit the company's website or call to ask which sweetener they use.

Get more from a daily aspirin. Take your aspirin at this time, and you will get the added benefit of lower blood pressure. In a Spanish study, people who took a 100 mg aspirin at bedtime for three months lowered their systolic blood pressure 6.8 points and diastolic blood pressure 4.6 points. People who took the same aspirin in the morning developed slightly higher blood pressure. Both groups got a more accurate measure of blood pressure than you get at your doctor's office because their blood pressure was monitored throughout the day and night.

Taking aspirin at night may help because the body systems that regulate blood pressure work differently at different times of day.

Sip your way to wide-open arteries. Tea may be the best beverage for your blood vessels. Drinking a cup of hibiscus tea three times a day lowered blood pressure nearly 6 points in six weeks in people with mild high blood pressure, one study reported. Studies suggest hibiscus relaxes blood vessels, acts as a diuretic, and reduces the activity of angiotensin converting enzyme (ACE) — like ACE inhibitor drugs for blood pressure.

Hibiscus is the main ingredient in Celestial Seasonings' caffeine-free Red Zinger and Lemon Zinger teas. You may also find it in other teas. To enjoy hibiscus tea, steep the tea bag in 8 ounces of hot water for six minutes.

If you've been drinking black tea instead of hibiscus, you haven't wasted your time. Black tea contains compounds that may keep your blood vessels flexible. In fact, an Australian study found that people who drank black tea three times a day for six months lowered their blood pressure 2 to 3 points.

Choose the safest NSAID for your heart

Many people turn to nonsteroidal anti-inflammatory drugs for pain relief, but these pills may raise your risk of heart attacks, strokes, and heart disease. Even worse, a new study reports some painkillers are harder on your heart than others.

The prescription painkiller rofecoxib (Vioxx) is the most dangerous, researchers warn. But indomethacin (Indocin) is also alarming, because it carries a combination of risks to your heart, digestive system, and nervous system.

The safest medicine for your heart and blood vessels is prescription or nonprescription naproxen (Aleve, Naprosyn). Low-dose ibuprofen (Motrin, Nuprin, Advil) is a close second as long as you take 1,200 milligrams (mg) or less a day. Naproxen and ibuprofen can still cause stomach bleeding and may interfere with the blood-thinning ability of low dose aspirin, so talk to your doctor about which is best for you.

Avoid unnecessary high blood pressure spikes. Your blood pressure is slightly above normal if it's between 120/80 and 140/90. Doctors call this prehypertension. If you have prehypertension, it's not just salt that you must manage to prevent rising blood pressure. Reducing salt only helps 60 percent of people with high blood pressure. But regardless of whether subtracting salt helps you, avoiding unnecessary spikes in your blood pressure may contribute to your good health and longevity. Consider making a few changes to protect yourself.

- Keep your bedroom warm. Research suggests a cold room means higher morning blood pressure, even with extra blankets and clothing to keep warm.

- Sing or listen to music, especially when facing stressful situations.

- Take a nap. People who took a one-hour nap had less of a spike in blood pressure when faced with a stressful task, a study found.

- Swim for your life. In a recent study of 43 adults ages 50 to 80, those swimming at least 15 minutes three or four days a week lowered their blood pressure from 131 to 122 mmHg in 12 weeks.

- Cut back on added sugars. Research shows you can lower your blood pressure by limiting foods with added sugars and drinks sweetened with sugar or high-fructose corn syrup.

- Get a good night's sleep. Men with normal blood pressure were much more likely to develop high blood pressure if they spent very little time in "slow-wave" or deep sleep. Those same people were not sleeping well due to problems like awakening several times a night, not sleeping long enough, or having sleep apnea. See the *Best ways to beat fatigue and boost energy* chapter for advice on getting a good night's sleep.

Discover the secret to any successful recipe

Spices can add delicious flavor to your meals, and as a bonus, many are rich in antioxidants.

Enjoy perfect seasoning without salt, and your blood pressure may benefit.

This handy chart spells out the best herbs and spices for flavoring fish, meats, sauces, vegetables, and more.

Spice	Use in	How it helps
basil	fish, poultry, veal, beef, potatoes, tomatoes, zucchini, green beans, soups, stews, tomato sauces, Spanish dishes	contains magnesium to help battle high blood pressure
chives	lean meats, potatoes, soups, sauces, Chinese dishes	may help prevent hip osteoarthritis
cilantro	salsa, pasta, Mexican or Chinese dishes	helps fight bacteria that cause food poisoning
dill	fish, chicken, soups, cabbage, cucumbers, green beans, carrots, German dishes	contains magnesium which may help prevent osteoporosis
fennel	fish, Italian or German dishes	may have antibacterial and anti-inflammatory effects
garlic	fish, lean meats, chicken, lamb, vegetables, soups, sauces, legumes, Italian or Greek dishes	may help battle colds, high blood pressure, cholesterol, and triglycerides
marjoram	fish, chicken, turkey, hamburger, eggplant, broccoli, potatoes, peas, zucchini, tomato sauce, tomato soup, French and Caribbean dishes	contains compounds that may help prevent cancer
oregano	fish, hamburgers, chicken, veal, soups, tomato sauce, broccoli, mushrooms, cabbage, zucchini, Italian, Greek, or Mexican dishes	may help lower risk of heart disease
parsley	fish, chicken, lean meats, vegetables, soups, sauces, Italian or Caribbean dishes	good source of vitamin K to help prevent osteoporosis and fractures
rosemary	fish, chicken, lamb, turnips, sauces, cauliflower, potatoes, French or Greek dishes	helps prevent cancer-causing compounds in meats
sage	lean meats, fish, poultry, broccoli, cauliflower, mushrooms, cabbage, stews, Mexican dishes	may help improve mood and mental ability
thyme	fish, lean meats, onions, soups, sauces, Caribbean recipes	has antibacterial powers

Defend your heart with a seafood supper

Vacation in Florida, New England, or even the Rocky Mountains, and you'll probably eat at least one delectable meal with fresh local fish — a tasty treat you won't soon forget. Fortunately, this is one vacation habit your doctor hopes you take home with you. Research suggests eating the right kind of fish regularly can help you blast away blood clots and reduce your chance of a heart attack.

To put this advantage to work for you, start eating fatty fish like salmon that are high in omega-3 fatty acids. Research suggests omega-3 fats like eicosapentaenoic acid (EPA) and docosahexaenoic acid (DHA) can do your heart worlds of good. In fact, studies of more than 30,000 people found that omega-3 fatty acids can help reduce your risk of a heart attack, even if you already have heart disease.

Experts suggest 500 milligrams (mg) of combined EPA and DHA daily may help prevent heart disease, and they recommend 800 to 1,000 mg a day to help prevent a heart attack or stroke if you have heart disease. Fortunately, eating two 3-ounce servings of fatty fish a week may help you reach 500 mg — or more. But if you've tried cooking fish, you may have hit a few stumbling blocks that have prevented you from enjoying seafood regularly. Try solutions like these to help you fall in love with fish again.

Know all your heart-healthy options. Can't afford salmon or just don't like it? Rainbow trout is a much cheaper fish that has all the same amazing health benefits. For example, a 3-ounce serving of either rainbow trout or sockeye salmon will deliver more than 1,000 mg of omega-3. That provides the full amount of omega-3 protection for existing heart disease in a small serving of fish about the size of a deck of cards. Both salmon and rainbow trout are also good sources of protein, selenium, niacin, and vitamin B12.

Of course, experts encourage you to eat a wide variety of fish that are rich in omega-3, so don't stop at rainbow trout. Other fish high in omega-3 fats include canned salmon, canned Pacific sardines, sablefish from Canada or Alaska, Atlantic mackerel from Canada, and smoked cisco. One 3-ounce serving of any of these can deliver more than 1,000 mg of omega-3 goodness.

Lower your risk of contamination. Visit any seafood restaurant in the southeastern states, and you'll probably see people enjoying their fish with a tall glass of iced tea. That's not a bad idea. Seafood can contain contaminants like mercury that can raise your risk of health problems.

But a recent laboratory study suggests that drinking coffee, green tea, or black tea may help your body absorb up to 60 percent less mercury from fish. More research is needed, and you should still aim to eat low-mercury fish like the ones listed above. But it wouldn't hurt to enjoy your fish dinner with a cup of tea or coffee just in case.

Banish fishy smells from your kitchen. Nobody wants a kitchen that smells like raw fish, so use this easy trick to wipe out odors naturally without chemical sprays. Boil vinegar in a pan on the stove, and open a few windows or doors for cross ventilation. You can also wash your fishy-smelling pans and utensils in vinegar and water, or rub them with a cut lemon. That should remove the fishy odor.

Learn to tell when fish is really done. Overcooking fish is easy, especially if you use rules like "fish is done when it flakes" or "cook 10 minutes for every inch of thickness." These rules are good for some fish, but they often allow too much moisture to escape during cooking.

So try this instead. Check whether the fish is done when it has cooked about eight minutes per inch of thickness. To see whether the center of the fish is translucent (still raw) or opaque (cooked), choose an inconspicuous spot on the fish, slide a knife in, and lift up part of the fish far enough to see its center. If you meet slight resistance when pulling the fish away from the bone, that's a good sign.

If you see a tiny bit of translucency at the center, remove the fish from the heat. The fish will continue to cook through and will be ready in a couple of minutes.

Buy from seasoned seafood sellers. For quality fresh fish, buy yours from a fish market or supermarket seafood counter where the staff is knowledgeable and understands how to handle fresh fish properly. Seafood inspectors say follow your nose to tell whether you've found a quality fish seller. If you wrinkle your nose at the fishy smell, shop somewhere else because the fish are no longer fresh. But if the area smells like an ocean breeze, and the staff can answer your questions, you've found the right place.

Turbocharge heart protection during weight loss

While you're trying to shed pounds, include lots of fish in your diet, and you'll be doing your heart a favor as well.

A study of obese Alaskan Yup'ik Eskimos found that those with high levels of omega-3 in their blood had normal levels of triglycerides and C-reactive protein (CRP), a marker of inflammation. Yet obese Yup'ik Eskimos who had the lowest levels of omega-3 had higher triglycerides and CRP, just like many other obese Americans. This puts them more at risk for heart disease.

On average, Yup'ik Eskimos take in far more omega-3 fats from fish than people in the lower 48 states. More research is needed to see if the Eskimos' high-fish diet is protective for everyone. But it's a good reason to enjoy an extra serving or two of fish each week.

5 danger signals you shouldn't ignore

Some seemingly harmless symptoms can sometimes be warning signs of heart trouble. Don't wait until you have a heart attack to find out about them. Recognizing these five problems could save your life.

Examine that acid indigestion. You had a great evening out with friends celebrating Cinco de Mayo, but now all that Mexican food seems to be giving you heartburn. Your chest feels as if a heavy weight is resting on it or feels squeezed tight and uncomfortable. Don't be so quick to dismiss this as heartburn, especially if the pain seems to be spreading to your arms, neck, jaw, shoulder, or back. You could be suffering from angina or even a heart attack.

Angina is chest pain that happens when the blood flow to your heart is constricted or blocked. If that blood flow is blocked suddenly, you may have a heart attack. Restoring that flow as quickly as possible could make the difference between life and death.

Seek emergency medical help if you suddenly start having unexplained chest pain, or if you already have episodes of angina but they change or come on with less exertion, occur during rest, become more severe, don't improve with rest or medicine, or accompany other heart attack symptoms.

Notice when you're out of breath. You buy a few light bags of groceries on your way home, but by the time you carry them halfway across the parking lot, you're out of breath or feel like you can't breathe properly. Maybe you even feel a tightness in your chest.

You assume you're just out of shape, but be careful. Shortness of breath and feeling tired all the time are common symptoms of heart failure. Your heart doesn't stop, like in a heart attack, but it also can't pump enough blood. This triggers fluid buildup in your lungs, making it harder to breathe. Shortness of breath and fatigue may also be signs of a heart attack.

Call 911 if shortness of breath comes on suddenly, is severe, or is accompanied by fainting, chest pain, nausea, or other signs of heart attack or heart failure.

Pay attention to swollen feet and ankles. You've noticed swelling in your feet and ankles and maybe even your legs. This problem may be caused by antidepressants, steroids, some blood pressure drugs, or another medication you take. But this type of swelling is also a common sign of heart failure, and can be a sign of liver failure or kidney failure. Call 911 if your swollen feet and ankles are accompanied by shortness of breath or chest pain. You should also seek medical help if:

- the swelling gets worse, and you have heart disease or kidney disease.

- you have a swollen leg that is red and warm to the touch.

- you start running a fever.

- you've had liver disease, and the swelling is spreading into your legs or torso.

Watch out for irregular heartbeats. Your heart may flutter or skip a beat when you fall in love, or it may race when you exercise, watch a horror movie, or feel any strong emotion. That's normal. But if you suddenly develop a racing heart, slowed heartbeat, irregular heartbeat, skipped beats, extra beats, or a flutter in your chest, these are arrhythmias.

Many arrhythmias are harmless, but some arrhythmias can make your heart stop beating, or may be a sign of a weakened or damaged heart. Arrhythmias are more likely to be dangerous if you already have heart disease or a faulty heart valve, or if your risk for heart disease is higher than average. Call your doctor if any of these apply to you:

- Your pulse is over 100 beats a minute.

- You've never had any kind of irregular heartbeat or unexplained racing heart before.

- You notice a change in your typical irregular heartbeats.

- You have extra heartbeats coming in groups of three more than six times a minute.

- You have high cholesterol, high blood pressure, or other risk factors for heart disease.

Call 911 if your arrhythmia lasts longer than a few minutes or is accompanied by near-fainting or by any heart attack or heart failure symptoms.

Beware of daytime sleepiness and loud snoring. Your spouse has long complained about your snoring, and lately you seem to be sleepy all the time. You struggle to stay awake while watching TV, reading, and even while stuck in traffic jams. This is not a sign of a heart attack, but you may have sleep apnea, and that affects your heart disease risk.

Sleep apnea is a condition where you stop breathing many times each night for 10 seconds or longer, but you never remember it. It has been linked to a higher risk of heart attack, stroke, and heart failure, but getting treatment lowers your odds of dying from heart disease. Snoring alone is not a sign of sleep apnea, but see your doctor if you also experience these symptoms:

- frequent or overwhelming daytime sleepiness

- irritability and hampered mental ability

- heartburn

- raucous snoring

- morning headaches

Fight back against the No. 1 killer of women

Heart attack symptoms for women are different than for men. So if you're a woman, how would you know if you're having a heart attack? One-third of women who have a heart attack have no chest pain, the most common symptom. But if you notice more subtle signs like these, you should still call 911 immediately.

- nausea, vomiting, or raging indigestion

- shortness of breath

- lightheadedness, dizziness, sudden fatigue, weakness, or breaking out in a cold sweat

- pain or discomfort in the arms, jaw, neck, back, or upper stomach

- pressure, squeezing, or pain in the center of your chest that lasts more than several minutes or lets up before coming back

Trans fats — the good, the bad, and the ugly

Trans fatty acids are often seen as the villain in the black cowboy hat, especially when it comes to heart health. But recent research has turned up a few surprises — some good, some bad, and some that are just plain ugly.

One may promote weight loss. Surprisingly, not all trans fats deserve to be called bad guys. Research suggests one trans fat in dairy products may play a positive role. Conjugated linoleic acid (CLA) appears to help boost your weight-loss efforts by reducing body fat. It's a naturally occurring trans fat, which is different from man-made.

Man-made trans fats are liquid oils turned into solid fats by a process called partial hydrogenation. They lurk in packaged foods, baked goods, and fried foods and are notorious for raising "bad" LDL cholesterol and lowering "good" HDL cholesterol. Natural trans fats in meats and dairy products are created by the stomach bacteria of cattle, sheep, or goats and may be less harmful.

That's not to say you should eat too much of them. A diet high in either natural or man-made trans fats raised LDL cholesterol, a Canadian study found. But a "moderate" diet with only 1.5 percent of calories from natural trans fats didn't change LDL or HDL cholesterol. That percentage would equal 30 calories from trans fats in a 2,000-calorie diet.

To avoid eating too many natural trans fats, some researchers suggest limiting saturated fats to 7 percent of daily calories because that helps limit trans fats, too. That's about 140 calories in a 2,000-calorie diet.

You may hear more about natural trans fats as manufacturers tout the benefits of CLA and work to boost its concentrations in milk and other dairy products.

Bad fats befuddle your brain. People with the highest blood levels of trans fats performed more poorly on tests of mental ability, and their brain scans revealed shrinking of the brain, an Oregon study found. Brain shrinking is associated with aging and dementia. To help prevent brain problems, switch from foods high in trans fats to foods like fish. Study participants who ate more fish performed better on tests of mental abilities, and their brain scans showed less shrinkage.

High amounts bring on the blues. Sunny Spain hardly seems like a place for depression. Yet a recent study found that Spanish people who ate high amounts of trans fats were nearly 50 percent more likely to develop depression than people who ate none.

But including more olive oil in your diet may lower the risk of depression, the researchers discovered. So replace trans fats with pesto and other olive oil dishes. To eat like the Spanish, try a Murcian salad with olives, tomatoes, roasted red peppers, green onions, tuna, and boiled egg, and top it with oil and vinegar salad dressing.

Stroke risk rises unless you take aspirin. Ischemic strokes, the kind from blocked blood vessels, account for 80 percent of strokes. Unfortunately, a study of 87,000 older women showed that women who ate the most trans fats raised their risk of ischemic strokes by 39 percent.

But aspirin may help. Out of a group of women who ate the most trans fats and took no aspirin, 66 percent had a higher risk of strokes. But women who ate the most trans fats and had been taking aspirin a long time saw no increase in stroke risk.

Of course, you should still watch your trans fat intake if you're on aspirin therapy. And if you don't already take aspirin, ask your doctor before you start. Daily aspirin can raise your risk of stomach bleeding.

7 simple steps to heart health

Make it to age 50 with ideal heart health, and you can probably live another 40 years free of heart disease and stroke. Experts from the American Heart Association outline what you need to do to achieve that ideal and live healthier longer.

- Never smoke, or have quit more than a year ago.

- Keep your body mass index (BMI) below 25.

- Do moderate physical activity like brisk walking at least 2 1/2 hours a week, or vigorous activity such as swimming laps at least 1 1/4 hours per week.

- Eat lots of fruits, vegetables, fish, and whole grains, and little sodium and sugar-sweetened beverages.

- Keep total cholesterol less than 200 mg/dL.

- Maintain blood pressure below 120/80 mmHg.

- Keep fasting blood glucose less than 100 mg/dL.

That sounds like a lot, but remember it's an ideal. Aim to get close.

Cancer risk may rise, too. Women who eat the most trans fats or have the most trans fats in their blood may have a higher risk of breast and ovarian cancer, European studies suggest. Eating trans fats may raise your risk of colon cancer, too.

They may tempt you to act "ugly." Eating trans fats was linked to aggressive behaviors and irritability in a recent study. If you've been worried about how easily you're tempted to become aggressive or have a moment of road rage, try eliminating trans fats from your diet. You may find life's daily problems much easier to take.

Labels hide the truth. According to U.S. Food and Drug Administration rules, any product that claims "zero trans fats" on the label can have up to 0.5 grams of trans fat per serving. Those tiny amounts add up.

Manufacturers are also replacing trans fats with saturated fats or with interesterified fats that may raise blood sugar and lower HDL cholesterol. Check the ingredient list, and avoid any "hydrogenated" products or saturated fats to stay safe.

Chow down on the perfect heart-smart breakfast

Fresh fruit and a crunchy wheat cereal with milk not only make the perfect breakfast, they can also help protect you from the No. 1 killer of both women and men — heart disease. This "silent" disease leads to more deaths in men than cancer, and more deaths in women than kidney disease and cancer combined. Fortunately, you can help prevent heart disease — or keep it from getting worse — by regularly enjoying the nutrients found in this delicious breakfast.

Get going with guava. Cube a cup of this tropical fruit, and protect yourself from cholesterol, homocysteine, and high blood pressure. Your heart will love this good news.

Studies have found that adding guava to your diet or eating extra guava helps lower your blood pressure and cholesterol. Fiber may be the reason why. That one cup of cubed guava delivers nearly 9 grams of fiber, more than a third of the daily value. And research suggests fiber can help lower blood pressure.

What's more, guava is a good source of the pectin fiber that helps lower cholesterol. For best results, enjoy your guava in the morning, and spruce up your snacks, lunch, and dinner with other good sources of pectin like apples, oranges, apricots, grapefruit, and carrots.

A cup of guava also delivers 80 micrograms of the B vitamin folate — 20 percent of the recommended value. You need folate to help control levels of the amino acid called homocysteine. Too much homocysteine in your bloodstream can damage your blood vessel walls. That damage raises your danger of heart attack and stroke.

Folate helps you fight back. Working with vitamins B6 and B12, folic acid helps convert homocysteine into amino acids that can be removed from your body. But you have to get enough folate to make a difference. Start with guava at breakfast, and add folate-rich foods like lentils, enriched rice, or pinto beans at lunch and dinner.

To pick the best guava for your morning meal, look for one with a pleasant fragrance. A ripe guava will give slightly if you press it gently. Wash your guava thoroughly before cutting or eating. You don't have to remove the seeds to enjoy this "poor man's apple of the tropics."

Fill up with hearty cereal. Cereal can make a difference to your heart because the food you eat can quickly affect your arteries. In a small study, researchers fed people two different breakfasts and measured how much their arteries widened or constricted after the meal. Eating a high-fiber, high-carbohydrate breakfast opened arteries by an astonishing 40 percent after just four hours. But eating a low-fiber meal of eggs, cheese, and sausage made arteries narrow and constrict, just as in previous studies with high-fat meals.

The study focused on people who had metabolic syndrome. That means they were overweight or obese and had two of the following risk factors for heart disease — high blood pressure, high triglycerides, low HDL cholesterol, or above-normal blood sugar. So even if you're not in perfect health, eating a high-fiber breakfast like this may help pave the way to free-flowing arteries.

The researchers suspect either the cereal fiber or powerful wheat bran antioxidants contributed to the good results. But they also point out that eating more cereal fiber has been linked to:

- a lower risk of heart disease and metabolic syndrome.

- lower odds of dying from heart disease.

- less of the body-wide inflammation that contributes to hardening of the arteries.

The researchers also suggest that regularly eating meals like the one in the study could help your arteries stay flexible throughout your life. And flexible arteries mean less risk of dying from heart disease.

To eat the same breakfast as the study participants, pour three-fourths to one cup of All-Bran Original cereal (or a similar high-fiber cereal) in a bowl, add about a cup of non-fat milk, spread jelly on whole-wheat toast, and top it off with a glass of cranberry juice. Make sure you eat enough cereal and whole-wheat toast to get 19 grams of fiber.

Add a cup of skim milk. Pour milk on your cereal to get a big boost of vitamin D. You could be 80 percent more likely to have a heart attack, stroke, or heart failure if you don't get enough of this important vitamin. In fact, a European study found that people with the lowest blood levels of vitamin D were more likely to die from heart disease within eight years than people with high vitamin D levels.

Fortified skim milk is a good place to start. A glass a day could help reduce inflammation and stress inside your blood vessels, and help you live longer.

Low vitamin D levels are also linked to high C-reactive protein (CRP), a sign of body-wide inflammation that can damage blood vessels. Low vitamin D levels have also been associated with a type of cell damage called oxidative stress, which is brought on by free radical molecules your body generates.

Blood vessel damage from body-wide inflammation and LDL-cholesterol damage from oxidative stress can help plaque build up inside your arteries, leading to hardening of the arteries. That raises your risk of heart attack, stroke, and heart failure. Fortunately, milk and other foods with vitamin D can help. Here's how.

- Getting enough vitamin D has been linked to lower levels of CRP and less inflammation. That's not just coincidence. One test tube study discovered that vitamin D reduces the levels of powerful inflammation-causing compounds found in your body.

- A Turkish study found that people with vitamin D deficiency who raised their vitamin D levels added flexibility to their arteries and reduced oxidized LDL cholesterol. Researchers concluded that vitamin D improved blood vessel flexibility by lowering oxidative stress.

Good sources of vitamin D include canned salmon, rainbow trout, canned light tuna, and foods fortified with vitamin D. But getting some of your vitamin D from skim milk may have extra benefits. When you drink skim milk, you may also be serving yourself a healthy portion of lower blood pressure.

A Spanish study found that people who enjoyed more servings of low-fat dairy products were less likely to get high blood pressure. Just two or three daily servings of common foods like skim milk and nonfat yogurt were enough to cut the incidence of high blood pressure in half.

Secret to lowering LDL faster

One well-known margarine spread claims it can start lowering your "bad" LDL cholesterol in two weeks, thanks to the spread's plant sterols. But what if you could do it in just six days? A new study suggests that's possible if you eat plant sterols several times a day instead of just once.

For six days, a group ate 1.8 grams of plant sterols at breakfast. In phase two, they divided the 1.8 grams between breakfast, lunch, and supper. Participants ate the same amount of plant sterols both times, but in the divided-dose phase, they lowered cholesterol by 6 percent. Eating the sterols once a day didn't lower cholesterol any more than eating no plant sterols.

Use sterol-fortified foods like margarine or orange juice to help divide your sterols among several meals. Eat 1.8 to 3 grams of plant sterols daily, and your cholesterol may drop faster, too.

Chocolate secrets for your heart and health

Talk about the perfect food. If there were a treat that could keep your heart and blood vessels in tiptop shape, plus make you look and feel better from head to toe, you would want to eat it every day, right? Make way for the tasty goodness of chocolate.

Provides heart-healthy benefits. Researchers did a review of previous studies about how chocolate can benefit heart risk factors. They looked at both short-term and long-term consumption of chocolate or cocoa, finding only good things like:

- lower blood pressure.

- increased flexibility of blood vessels to boost blood flow.

- better LDL and HDL cholesterol numbers.

- improved insulin resistance.

Previous researchers found that eating chocolate may even lower your risk of stroke. Experts think an antioxidant compound in cocoa, epicatechin, gets credit for its heart-healthy powers.

And just look at the other ways chocolate helps your health.

Good for your teeth. Believe it or not, natural chemicals in cocoa have the power to cut inflammation and protect your teeth against erosion and decay.

As a doctoral student at Tulane University, Arman Sadeghpour compared theobromine, a natural chemical in cocoa, with fluoride to see which had the strongest enamel-strengthening power. Theobromine was more protective than even fluoride, already used to protect your teeth.

Sadeghpour has now developed a toothpaste, called Theodent, that includes theobromine as the active ingredient. You can find it in select Whole Foods stores. You can also feel a little better about eating chocolate, although the benefits of theo-bromine may be undermined by the sugar in chocolate candy. So moderation is still key.

Makes your skin look better. You can try a facial mask containing cocoa to help your skin look and feel better, but science has shown how eating chocolate benefits skin as well.

Women in a study drank one-half cup of cocoa daily for 12 weeks. The drink contained the same amount of flavanols as a 3 1/2-ounce serving of dark chocolate. By the end of the study, their skin was less dry, scaly, and rough than at the start. They also noticed better blood flow in their skin, and more resistance to sun damage. In fact, their skin looked and felt better than the skin of women who drank a low-flavanol cocoa for that same 12 weeks.

Boosts your mood. You don't need researchers to tell you chocolate can cheer you up, but scientists have tackled this issue repeatedly anyway.

One study involved having stressed-out people eat 1 1/2 ounces of dark chocolate daily for two weeks, then have their levels of stress hormones tested. By the end, they were producing less cortisol and catecholamines, stress hormones expelled in urine.

Other experts have pointed out that cocoa powder contains compounds that boost the levels of endorphins and serotonin in your brain, leading to a better mood. And another study noted that people who are depressed tend to eat more chocolate than happy people, possibly because they are trying to self-medicate their way to a better mood.

May keep you slim. It sounds like a dream, but it's true. Researchers in San Diego studying statin use asked roughly 1,000 men and women completing questionnaires the question, "How many times a week do you consume chocolate?" They also recorded how much exercise they got and checked their weight by tracking body mass index (BMI).

On average, people in the study ate chocolate twice a week. The more often they indulged, the lower their BMI. Those who ate chocolate five times a week had a BMI about one point lower than people who ate no chocolate. That translates to about 5 to 8 pounds lighter, depending on height. Researchers found no relation between BMI and the amount of chocolate eaten each time. It was all about the frequency.

Of course, overindulgence is a problem since chocolate candy can be high in fat and sugar. Other researchers tackled that problem, and they discovered the best time to enjoy chocolate without encouraging cravings.

Turns out eating chocolate when you're hungry may lead to more cravings. In contrast, eating it 15 to 30 minutes after a meal may make you more satisfied and less likely to battle a craving. Indulge in a small chocolate dessert, and it may be all you need.

Basic cocoa brand takes the cake

The cooking experts at *Cook's Illustrated* magazine tested several brands of cocoa powder to see if a higher price guaranteed better taste. Their results were surprising.

The experts compared eight brands of cocoa powders, some common and some hard to find, looking for the best taste when used in cookies, cakes, and hot cocoa. They considered various features like fat content, particle size, and how the cocoa beans were roasted.

Judges said the winning brand — Hershey's Natural Cocoa Powder Unsweetened — had deep complexity and great chocolate flavor. It's easy to find at your grocery story and averages just over $7 per pound — much less than the luxury brands tested.

Sometimes an old standby is the best choice.

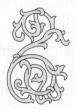

Osteoporosis: bone-building breakthroughs

Steer clear of bone-zapping foods

Common foods can suck the calcium right out of your bones. You probably eat and drink them every day, but they're easy to avoid if you know what to look for.

Set aside the saltshaker. Salty foods may wage an assault on your bones. That's because when your body tries to get rid of excess sodium through your urine, it flushes calcium along with it. One study found that a high-salt diet caused women to lose 36 percent more calcium than a low-salt diet. And boosting calcium intake didn't help.

A recent study of mice by researchers at the University of Alberta in Canada sheds some light on the link between sodium and calcium absorption. "We found a molecule that seems to have two jobs — regulating the levels of both calcium and sodium in the body," says lead researcher Todd Alexander.

"When the body tries to get rid of sodium via the urine, our findings suggest the body also gets rid of calcium at the same time. This is significant because we are eating more and more sodium in our diets, which means our bodies are getting rid of more and more calcium."

That's why it's important to cut your salt intake. The National Osteoporosis Foundation says that getting less than 2,400 milligrams (mg) of sodium a day shouldn't harm your bones.

Check the sodium content on a food's Nutrition Facts label, keeping in mind that if a serving contains 20 percent or more of your Daily Value, it's high in sodium. Also remember to account for the number of servings you plan to eat to get your true sodium intake.

Your best strategy is to limit prepackaged, processed, or canned foods, and go easy on the saltshaker during cooking and serving.

Curb the caffeine. Coffee and other caffeinated beverages give you a burst of energy, but they may also give your bones a jolt. Caffeine may cause your body to flush out more calcium through urine and stool. This can put you at risk for bone loss and fractures.

In the Framingham Osteoporosis Study, researchers found that over a 12-year period, drinking 2.5 units or more of caffeine a day raised the risk of hip fracture at each two-year health check. One cup of coffee equals one unit, while one cup of tea equals 0.5 units.

A recent Brazilian study found that rats who received caffeine showed more bone loss and slower bone healing following surgery.

But there is some good news. It seems you can counteract this effect by getting more calcium in your diet. Aim for 40 mg more calcium for every cup of coffee.

Cut down on cola. Soft drinks may soften your bones. That's what an analysis of participants in the Framingham study discovered. Women who regularly drank cola had lower bone mineral density (BMD) in their hips. The findings did not apply to men.

Caffeine could be partially to blame, but that's not the only factor. Those who drank decaffeinated sodas still had lower bone density, although not as low as the caffeinated soda drinkers.

Another possible factor is the phosphoric acid in carbonated colas. Getting too much phosphorus and too little calcium could lower the calcium levels in your blood. This stimulates the release of parathyroid hormone (PTH), which causes the body to pull calcium out of bones and into the blood to bring levels back up. Phosphoric acid may also block absorption of calcium from food.

Women who drank the most colas also got the least calcium every day, which could contribute to their low bone density. The occasional cola is probably fine, but you may not want to drink it regularly if you're worried about osteoporosis.

Stronger bones mean fewer scans

If you're 67 or older with a recent bone density T-score between -1.49 and 0, you can breathe a sigh of relief. You may not need another bone density scan for 15 years.

Researchers found it would take that long for osteoporosis to develop in just 10 percent of postmenopausal women with normal bone density or mild osteopenia. Women with moderate or advanced osteopenia need to be rechecked more often.

Medications that lower bone density, or changes in your health, may require more frequent scans. As always, follow your doctor's advice.

Avoid alcohol. Alcohol doesn't necessarily suck calcium from your bones, but it can harm them nonetheless — especially when you overdo it. Drinking three or more alcoholic beverages a day puts men at high risk for osteoporosis. Research shows that older women who drink heavily — six or more drinks a day — have greater bone loss than those who drink only occasionally.

Chronic heavy drinking, particularly early in life, compromises bone strength. It's not reversible, even if you stop drinking. Alcohol seems to decrease bone density and harm other properties, such as elasticity, stiffness, toughness, and ability to bear weight.

But alcohol may be helpful in moderation. An Oregon State study found that moderate alcohol consumption may offset bone loss associated with menopause. In the study, 40 post-menopausal women who normally had one or two drinks a day abstained from alcohol for two weeks. During that time, researchers noticed evidence of higher bone turnover, a risk factor for osteoporosis-related fractures. Less than one day after the women resumed drinking, their bone turnover rates returned to normal.

"Drinking moderately as part of a healthy lifestyle that includes a good diet and exercise may be beneficial for bone health, especially in postmenopausal women," says Oregon State researcher Urszula Iwaniec.

If you already enjoy an occasional drink, feel free to keep it up. But don't start drinking just to protect your bones. It may not help and could even harm them.

Bone density tests are not just for women

Around 600,000 men suffer osteoporosis-related fractures each year in the United States. That's like having every person in Boston walking around with a broken bone. It goes to show that osteoporosis is not just a women's problem — men are also at risk, especially as they get older.

And the condition can be more serious in men than in women, more likely ending in death after a serious fracture. New guidelines from experts at the Endocrine Society suggest men take these steps as they age to stay safe from osteoporosis-related fractures.

- Get a bone-density test using dual-energy X-ray absorptiometry (DXA) if you're 70 years or older. Consider having it if you're 50 to 69 years if you also have risk factors like low body weight, having already suffered a fracture, and smoking.

- Take vitamin D supplements if your levels are low.

- If you're 50 or older and have suffered a fracture of the spine or hip, consider drug treatment. Then have your doctor order a DXA every year or two to be sure treatment is working.

- Eat 1,000 to 1,200 milligrams (mg) of calcium daily, especially from foods.

But research in Australia found that exercise works best. Middle-age men in the study either drank milk, exercised, did both, or did neither. Milk drinkers got 1,000 mg of calcium and 800 international units (IU) of vitamin D daily from the beverage, and exercisers lifted weights and did activities like running three times a week.

After 18 months, men who exercised had about a 2-percent increase in bone density. Surprisingly, drinking milk didn't seem to help.

Unusual tips to strengthen your skeleton

You probably know that getting enough calcium in your diet helps guard your bones from osteoporosis. Strength training can also help ward off brittle bones and fractures. But you can go beyond the basics for an extra dose of protection. Bone up on these unexpected ways to strengthen your skeleton.

Try some turmeric. Turmeric has long been popular as a key spice in Indian, Chinese, and Indonesian cooking. But, thanks to recent research, it may become known as the spice that prevents bone loss. Credit goes to curcumin, a mighty anti-oxidant that gives turmeric its distinctive golden-orange color.

Bone loss speeds up after menopause. So studies looked at animals that have experienced the equivalent of menopause.

University of Arizona researchers tested two turmeric extracts similar to the turmeric supplements available to consumers. Both extracts contained curcuminoids — powerful natural compounds that may limit your body's population of bone-removing osteoclast cells. Fewer osteoclasts may mean less bone loss.

Curcuminoids made up only 41 percent of extract A, while they made up 94 percent of extract B. Animals who received extract B three times a week lost up to 50-percent less bone density than animals that didn't.

A recent Malaysian study found similar results. Curcumin treatment at high doses was as effective — but safer than — Premarin, an estrogen replacement therapy, for reversing bone changes in rats.

More studies are needed to determine whether turmeric works as well on people as it did for the study animals. Meanwhile, consider fitting more turmeric into your diet.

Start by adding a quarter teaspoon to your favorite foods like chili, pasta sauce, stew, curry, or sautéed vegetables. You can also spice up your hot chocolate, tomato juice, ketchup, and mustard. Increase the amount of turmeric according to your taste.

Sip yerba mate tea. Wash down all that turmeric with some tasty yerba mate tea. Made from a tropical plant, this tea is popular in South America but is also available in health food stores and online.

A study from Argentina suggests yerba mate tea has a protective effect on bone. The study included 146 postmenopausal women who drank at least four cups of yerba mate tea a day for four or more years and an equal number of women who did not drink yerba mate.

Yerba mate drinkers had a 9.7-percent higher bone mineral density (BMD) in the lumbar spine, or lower back, and a 6.2-percent higher BMD in the femoral neck, the thin area of the thigh bone right below your hip socket.

Keep in mind that yerba mate can be high in caffeine. Other studies have shown a negative effect of caffeine on bone density.

Pop some prunes. Prunes, or dried plums, are famous for keeping you regular. But making them a regular part of your diet may also help protect your bones.

In a Florida State University study, postmenopausal women who ate 100 grams of dried plums — about 10 prunes — a day for a year boosted the bone mineral density of their spines and elbow bones compared to women who ate the same amount of dried apples. Both groups also received calcium and vitamin D supplements.

"I have tested numerous fruits, including figs, dates, strawberries, and raisins, and none of them come anywhere close to having the effect on bone density that dried plums, or prunes, have," says Florida State professor Bahram H. Arjmandi. "All fruits and vegetables have a positive effect on nutrition, but in terms of bone health, this particular food is exceptional."

The study also found evidence that the women who ate dried plums had lower rates of bone breakdown. Arjmandi believes this is why bone density improved.

If you can't stand the thought of eating whole dried plums, chop them finely, and mix them into rice like raisins, or add them to baked goods.

Exercise turns stem cells into bone

Remember how Rumpelstiltskin used his magic spindle to turn straw into gold? Aerobic exercise — activities like running and swimming — may offer the same kind of "magical" transformation to benefit your bones.

Researchers at McMaster University in Canada compared mice who exercised with those forced to live like couch potatoes. The exercisers ran on a treadmill for less than an hour, three times a week.

After 10 weeks of workouts, the researchers found exercising mice had developed more bone cells and fewer fat cells than sedentary mice. Mesenchymal stem cells in their bone marrow could have gone either way, but exercise triggered more bone cell production.

That's good news if you'd rather run than lift weights. Your bones win either way.

Get enough sleep. Weeks or months of getting less sleep than you should can be bad news for bones, an animal study suggests. Researchers discovered that chronic sleep loss led to less formation of new bone without reducing the removal of old bone. Naturally, this lowered bone mineral density.

If chronic sleep loss causes the same effects in people, it may lead to the faulty bone processes associated with osteoporosis. In addition, your body may have a harder time repairing the microscopic bone damage caused by your normal activities. These problems may reduce bone healing after surgery and raise your risk of fractures.

If you rarely get enough slumber, sleeping more may help save your skeleton. If you have trouble sleeping, see the chapter *Best ways to beat fatigue and boost energy* for drug-free ideas that can help.

Seek out more vitamin C. Vitamin D is not the only vitamin that boosts bones. "The medical world has known for some time that low amounts of vitamin C can cause scurvy and brittle bones, and that higher vitamin C intake is associated with higher bone mass in humans," says Mone Zaidi, MD, professor of medicine at the Mount Sinai School of Medicine and director of the Mount Sinai Bone Program.

To find out whether vitamin C could also protect against bone loss in older women, Zaidi's research group compared three groups of mice. The first group underwent surgery that mimics menopause and promotes bone loss. The second group also had the surgery, but received high daily doses of vitamin C. The third "control" group did not have surgery. After eight weeks, the first group had significantly lower bone density than the control group, but the vitamin C group had roughly the same bone density as the control group.

"What this study shows is that large doses of vitamin C, when ingested orally by mice, actively stimulate bone formation to protect the skeleton," Zaidi says. It may do this by prompting immature osteoblast cells to become fully mature osteoblasts that can build bone. These osteoblasts may build more new bone fast enough to help prevent bone loss, he explains.

"Further research may discover that dietary supplements may help prevent osteoporosis in humans," says Zaidi. But first, new studies must find out whether vitamin C has the same effect in humans as in mice. Meanwhile, make sure you get enough vitamin C by eating foods like sweet peppers, oranges, papayas, strawberries, and broccoli.

Opt for olive oil. Heart-healthy olive oil may be good for bones, a Spanish study suggests. This study assigned older men to one of three diets:

- a Mediterranean diet enriched with olive oil.

- a Mediterranean diet enriched with nuts.

- a low-fat diet.

After the men followed their diets for two years, the researchers checked their blood for compounds like osteocalcin and other "bone markers." Higher levels of bone markers may mean you are making more bone. Only the men who ate the diet enriched with olive oil had increased bone markers. That may be reason enough to "bone up" on delicious Mediterranean recipes with olive oil.

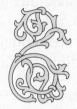

Eye problems: see your way to clearer vision

5 tricks to perk up tired eyes

You finally did it — spent the past three hours learning to post videos to Facebook and read your granddaughter's Twitter feeds on the computer. Then you blogged about your success and sent emails to your 20 closest friends. But now your eyes are tired and red, and they feel too dry and sore to enjoy your newfound computer skills.

Eyes can feel tired and overworked for many reasons other than too much time staring at a video monitor. Try these remedies to make your peepers feel peppy.

Keep eyeglasses pristine. Keep a sharp eye on how clean your eyeglass lenses are so you don't have to squint to see through a layer of oil and dirt.

The best way to clean your glasses is to first get them wet by rinsing under lukewarm water. Your eyeglasses will last longer if you do this before cleaning them, since it washes away grit that could cause scratches. Then use a mild dish-washing liquid without lotion, perhaps something like Dawn. Put a few drops on your clean fingers, then rub gently on both sides of the lenses. Rinse again with lukewarm water.

Dry your eyeglasses with a clean, lint-free towel that's 100-percent cotton. Never use a paper towel, tissue, or other paper product, since these can scratch your lenses.

Enjoy your morning coffee. New research shows caffeine may reduce the symptoms of dry eye syndrome. This condition makes your eyes feel scratchy and dry, and it can interfere with your vision. It affects about 4 million people in the United States, mostly older folks. Treatments include eye washes, artificial tears, and warm compresses.

A study in Japan involved giving people caffeine pills, then measuring their tear production. All 78 people who took caffeine had significantly greater tear production within 45 minutes, so they didn't have to wait long for relief. But they took a pretty large dose of caffeine, about equal to the amount in four or five cups of regular coffee.

Experts aren't sure exactly how caffeine helps, but they suspect it stimulates tear glands to produce more tears. Caffeine is known to increase other secretions, such as digestive juices and saliva.

The researchers also noticed different effects based on different genetic markers, or heredity. That's why they think the remedy might work best on people who are more sensitive to caffeine's effects. But if your family history includes glaucoma, you may want to be more cautious about your coffee intake. See the box on the next page.

Too much coffee may raise glaucoma risk

Scandinavians drink the most caffeinated coffee and also have the highest rate of exfoliation glaucoma. Researchers were interested in whether there was a link between the two.

They looked at more than 120,000 people from the Nurses' Health Study and Health Professionals Follow-up Study, who had completed questionnaires about what they drank and their eye health.

Turns out people who drank three or more cups of caffeinated coffee daily had a higher risk of developing this type of -. There was no link with other caffeinated beverages, like tea or colas. The risk of eye disease was especially great for women with a family history of glaucoma.

It's still too early to make real recommendations about coffee drinking. If other researchers find similar results, then a family history of glaucoma may turn out to be a warning to limit your daily coffee habit.

Consider flaxseed oil supplements. Your tears are more than just saltwater. They also contain oil, mucus, proteins, and antibodies. That may explain why the oil you eat can affect your tears and improve dry eye syndrome.

Researchers found that people who took up to 9,000 milligrams (mg) daily of flaxseed oil supplements noticed improvement in their dry eye symptoms after three months.

That's a pretty big dose of flaxseed oil, so people started by taking smaller doses. Too much flaxseed oil can bring on side effects like diarrhea.

Flaxseed oil is rich in omega-3 fatty acids — the same type of healthy fats that are good for your heart. Some experts say a typical Western diet, containing lots of omega-6 fatty acids and not enough omega-3, can reduce the amount of oil secreted from the glands in your eyelids. Flaxseed oil helps create softer secretions from your oil glands, so oil can be released to help the flow of tears.

Taking supplements of omega-3 fish oil might also work to relieve dry eyes, and they might be easier to tolerate than flaxseed oil.

Blink, take a break, lower the brightness. Remember these three B's, and your eyes won't beg for attention after a session on the computer.

- Remember to blink frequently. Typically you blink less often when you stare at a computer screen, making your eyes feel dry and tired. Blinking lets tears bathe your eyes to help them feel more comfortable.

- Take breaks fairly often, again allowing your eyes to relax.

- Lower the brightness of your computer monitor. You can also buy a screen made to cut down glare on your computer monitor. This may help if lower-tech solutions don't do the trick.

Save your tea bags. Chrysanthemums are an ancient secret for tired eyes. Some people swear by placing the flower heads of chrysanthemums on their closed eyelids to ease overstrained eyes.

The tea works, too, but not necessarily by drinking it. Instead, take two used wet chrysanthemum tea bags, and place one on each closed eyelid. Leave in place for five minutes.

Antioxidants in chrysanthemum tea are believed to relax your blood vessels, ease irritation, and soothe your eyes. The relaxing treatment may even reduce under-eye circles and make your eyes look less puffy.

Surprising habits that put your vision at risk

It's easy to take good eyesight for granted. But when you let other parts of your body go to pot, your eyes may soon follow. Don't let these bad health habits steal your clarity of vision.

Passing by the fish counter. Pop open a can of tuna, and fill your freezer with salmon. These tasty fish can slash your risk of vision-stealing macular degeneration.

Researchers in Australia found that people who tended to eat fish once a week had a 40-percent lower risk of developing age-related macular degeneration (AMD) than those who rarely ate it, while those who ate fish three times a week cut their risk by an astounding 75 percent.

The healthy omega-3 fatty acids in fatty fish get the credit. Experts believe they fight inflammation in your body, protecting cells in your retina.

Leaving your sunglasses at home. People with blue eyes have a higher risk of both cataracts and AMD. Less pigment means more sunlight can get into your eyes to do damage. Too much sun can lead to photokeratitis, like a sunburn of your corneas, along with skin cancer on your eyelids and the growth of vision-blocking spots on the whites of your eyes.

That's why it's important to protect your eyes from the sun, just as you protect your skin with sunblock. Your best bet is wearing sunglasses. But not all sunglasses are created equal. Look for a pair with these traits:

- lenses with both UVA and UVB protection of at least 95 percent.

- wraparound styles to keep out light from the sides.

- the right tint. Don't confuse darkness with tint, since lenses that look darker may not actually be blocking more light. Your eyes can be fooled by lenses that only seem dark. They can let your pupils open up to allow you to see, letting in more light and thus doing more damage. Look for gray, amber, brown, or green lenses that block at least 80 percent, but no more than 92 percent, of transmissible light.

Cheap sunglasses — a bargain for your eyes

When it comes to buying a pair of quality sunglasses, sometimes cheaper is just as good. Focus on getting the eye-protection features you need rather than assuming you have to pay a lot.

Dr. Lee Duffner, an ophthalmologist in sunny Florida, says the best pair could very well be a bargain.

"It's not really price-related," he says. "I've seen very expensive sunglasses that are not good ultraviolet absorbers, and I've seen cheap sunglasses that were great ultraviolet absorbers."

But avoid the cheapest-of-the-cheap — sunglasses from sidewalk vendors. You can find a decent pair for less than $20 at a reputable drugstore.

Getting lazy about belly fat. It's bad for your heart, and it's also bad for your eyes if you're a man.

Researchers measured how much abdominal fat middle-age and older people carried, then checked to see how many developed age-related macular degeneration. This eye disease is a leading cause of blindness among older people.

The study found that men had a 13-percent higher risk of developing early-stage AMD for every 0.1 increase in their waist-to-hip ratio. In other words, being bigger in the middle meant a greater chance of AMD. Even worse, the same amount of belly fat correlated with a 75-percent greater risk of the more severe late-stage AMD.

But this was not the case for women. Instead, a bit of belly fat correlated with a slightly lower risk of developing AMD among women in the study. Abdominal fat releases estrogen, which researchers suspect may be protective in women but not in men.

Using the tiny juice glasses. Upsize to a larger serving of orange juice every morning, and protect your precious eyesight as you age.

Studies have shown that getting more antioxidant vitamins in your diet — vitamin C in particular — may cut your risk of cataracts. Both nuclear and cortical cataracts were less common among people getting lots of vitamin C from food and supplements.

The Blue Mountains Eye Study followed people in Australia for 10 years, tracking what they ate and what supplements they took. Those who ate lots of vitamin C–rich foods like citrus fruits and juices and cruciferous vegetables seemed to be especially well protected.

Experts already knew that oxidative stress, or free radical damage to the lens of your eye, is a risk factor for cataracts. So it makes sense that an antioxidant powerhouse like vitamin C could prevent cataracts from forming.

And another study found that women who tend to eat a balanced diet — staying close to the food pyramid's variety of fruits, vegetables, whole grains, and so on — have a lower risk of cataracts.

Letting your blood pressure go its own way. It's important to follow your doctor's orders when it comes to keeping control of high blood pressure.

People with high blood pressure have a greater risk of developing neovascular age-related macular degeneration, also known as wet AMD. Having high levels of C-reactive protein, a measure of inflammation in your body, also means you're at a higher risk.

Wet AMD is the major cause of AMD-related vision loss. It occurs when new blood vessels are formed within the eye, and they leak fluid and blood under the retina. This can lead to scar tissue forming, replacing light-sensitive cells that are needed to see properly.

Experts also have noticed a higher risk of developing glaucoma for people battling heart disease and high blood pressure. So follow a heart-healthy lifestyle, and see if it may also protect your vision.

Popping aspirin like it's candy. Your doctor may have you taking a daily aspirin to fend off heart disease. But researchers in the Netherlands found that seniors who take daily aspirin are twice as likely to suffer from AMD as people who don't take aspirin.

The study looked at nearly 5,000 people older than 65 in countries all over Europe. The link was only to the wet form of AMD, not the dry form, and only to late-stage AMD.

But experts warn that perfect eyesight won't do you much good if you are dying from heart disease, so follow your doctor's advice regarding daily aspirin therapy.

Steering clear of your eye doctor. You know you should go. But the National Health Interview Survey found that 40 percent of adults with severe visual impairment and half of those with at least some eye problems had not seen an eye-care specialist in the previous 12 months.

Regular eye checkups are especially important if you're older than 65, since getting older is related to many sight-stealing conditions like glaucoma, macular degeneration, and cataracts. It's also important to see an eye doctor if you have diabetes, so you can avoid vision loss from diabetic retinopathy.

With screening and care by an ophthalmologist or optometrist covered by Medicare, there's really no reason not to go. The annual preventive and diagnostic tests covered by Medicare include checks for glaucoma and macular degeneration, both treatable conditions.

Be your own optician

You can save hundreds on reading glasses by buying a perfectly good pair for $3 off the rack at the drugstore. These basic magnifying glasses work fine for short periods of time — unless you have astigmatism or other vision problems. Here's how to fit the plastic frames to your face.

- Using a hair dryer, heat up the arms of the eyeglasses for about 15 to 20 seconds.

- Bend the frame slightly at the temple to even out the arms. If one ear is higher than the other, you can make your glasses sit evenly.

- Bend both arms inward just a bit to make your glasses tighter. Bend them outward to loosen the fit.

- Once the fit is just right, hold your eyeglasses under cold running water for a few seconds to set the new shape.

Novel ways to regain perfect eyesight

Benjamin Franklin gets credit for inventing bifocals to help middle-age people cope with age-related vision changes. But that was more than 200 years ago, and scientists are still coming up with ways to help you see better. Check out these three innovations.

Treat lazy eyes with video games. Eye doctors used to think amblyopia, or lazy eye, had to be corrected before about age eight by placing a patch over the stronger eye. After that age, it might be too late to fix. Adults with lazy eye were thought to be out in the cold.

But a small study tested playing video games to treat lazy eye in adults. The idea was that by patching the dominant eye while people used the "lazy" eye to focus on the game, they might quickly train that eye to function properly.

And it worked. After just 40 hours of game-playing, the 20 people in the study showed improved visual acuity and three-dimensional perception. They played either Medal of Honor Pacific Assault — a first-person shooting game — or SimCity Societies, a non-action game. People in a control group had their dominant eyes patched while they focused on activities like watching television, knitting, and surfing the Internet. They showed no significant change during this phase but improved substantially in the video-game phase.

The game therapy worked five times faster than traditional patch therapy used with children. It was a small study, but the researchers say it shows promise that the adult brain has enough plasticity to improve amblyopia.

Get eye medicine via contact lenses. Putting drops in your eyes can be difficult and uncomfortable, and sometimes the medicine doesn't even end up where it needs to be. In fact, within about five minutes of using glaucoma medicine eye drops, the medicine is gone. It moves away from your eye via tears, circulating through the bloodstream and causing side effects.

That's why experts are working on contact lenses that can dispense medicine. One method involves lenses loaded with vitamin E and glaucoma medicine. The vitamin E creates "transport barriers" that hold the medicine in your eye. Early research shows vitamin E helps medicine stay in contact with your eye for 100 times as long as when other types of lenses are used. More research is needed before the vitamin E lenses will be available.

Another new option is a hydrogel lens that can hold medicine in your eye for 30 days or more. Researchers expect to be able to change the rate of drug delivery by altering the makeup of the lens. Ultimately, a lens that delivers medicine for as long as 100 days may be available.

Cataracts? Select your bionic eyes. If you need cataract surgery to replace a lens that's become clouded, you get to choose what kind of intraocular lens (IOL) implant you want. IOLs come in two basic types.

Monofocal (fixed focus) lenses let you choose between great vision at near, middle, or far distances.

Some people have one eye fitted with a near-vision lens, and the other fitted with a distance-vision lens. With this type of monovision, your brain should be able to adjust, letting you see well both near and far. But some folks have trouble getting used to it. You'll probably have better vision after surgery for reading or driving at night with monofocal lenses, but you may still need to wear glasses.

The cost of basic monofocal lenses is covered by Medicare or health insurance. But if you choose to upgrade to a special toric lens to correct astigmatism, it's probably not covered.

Multifocal or accommodative lenses can correct your vision at all distances.

- A multifocal lens is made of several concentric rings, each with a different power of correction to help you see better at near, middle, and far distances. Eighty-five percent of people who choose these lenses don't need glasses for distance or near activities. The downside is you may see some halos or rings around lights at night, and you may lose some contrast in vision.

- Accommodative lenses work by letting your eye muscles position the lens for best vision, depending on how close or far you are looking. These function best when implanted in both eyes.

Neither multifocal nor accommodative lenses are covered by Medicare. You'll probably pay the difference in price, or around $1,500 to $2,500 per eye.

Other options being developed include a lens with a slight yellow tint to filter out harmful blue light waves that can damage your retina. You won't see a color difference, but the lenses will protect your retina just as your own lens did before cataract surgery.

Cataract surgery a boon to your brain

Keep an eye on vision changes, and you just may keep your brain sharp as well. People with Alzheimer's disease (AD) can get extra benefits from surgery to remove a cataract.

Researchers identified 38 people suffering from both AD and cataracts. After cataract surgery, all but one person in the study enjoyed improved distance and near vision.

Three months later researchers checked the cognitive abilities of these AD sufferers. For a quarter of the group, the ability to think and interact with the world had improved. Many had less depression, and they slept better. These are the same changes expected in people without dementia after cataract surgery.

Previous research found that people who regularly visit an eye doctor and have their poor vision treated are less likely to develop dementia as they age. All the more reason to take good care of your eyes.

INDEX